Exploring Early Childhood Care and Education Levers to Improve Population Health

PROCEEDINGS OF A WORKSHOP

Theresa M. Wizemann, *Rapporteur*

Roundtable on Population Health Improvement

Board on Population Health and Public Health Practice

Health and Medicine Division

The National Academies of
SCIENCES · ENGINEERING · MEDICINE

THE NATIONAL ACADEMIES PRESS
Washington, DC
www.nap.edu

THE NATIONAL ACADEMIES PRESS 500 Fifth Street, NW Washington, DC 20001

This activity was supported by contracts between the National Academy of Sciences and Aetna Foundation (#10002892), The California Endowment (#10003309), Dartmouth-Hitchcock Medical Center, Fannie E. Rippel Foundation, Health Resources and Services Administration (DHHS-10003351), Kaiser East Bay Community Foundation (#10002957), The Kresge Foundation (#10002910), Nemours, New York State Health Foundation (#10001272), New York University Langone Medical Center, Office of the Assistant Secretary for Health (#10003388), Robert Wood Johnson Foundation (#10001270), Samueli Institute, and Wake Forest Baptist Medical Center. Any opinions, findings, conclusions, or recommendations expressed in this publication do not necessarily reflect the views of any organization or agency that provided support for the project.

International Standard Book Number-13: 978-0-309-47683-6
International Standard Book Number-10: 0-309-47683-6
Digital Object Identifier: https://doi.org/10.17226/25129

Additional copies of this publication are available for sale from the National Academies Press, 500 Fifth Street, NW, Keck 360, Washington, DC 20001; (800) 624-6242 or (202) 334-3313; http://www.nap.edu.

Printed in the United States of America

Suggested citation: National Academies of Sciences, Engineering, and Medicine. 2019. *Exploring early childhood care and education levers to improve population health: Proceedings of a workshop*. Washington, DC: The National Academies Press. doi: https://doi.org/10.17226/25129.

The National Academies of

SCIENCES • ENGINEERING • MEDICINE

The **National Academy of Sciences** was established in 1863 by an Act of Congress, signed by President Lincoln, as a private, nongovernmental institution to advise the nation on issues related to science and technology. Members are elected by their peers for outstanding contributions to research. Dr. Marcia McNutt is president.

The **National Academy of Engineering** was established in 1964 under the charter of the National Academy of Sciences to bring the practices of engineering to advising the nation. Members are elected by their peers for extraordinary contributions to engineering. Dr. C. D. Mote, Jr., is president.

The **National Academy of Medicine** (formerly the Institute of Medicine) was established in 1970 under the charter of the National Academy of Sciences to advise the nation on medical and health issues. Members are elected by their peers for distinguished contributions to medicine and health. Dr. Victor J. Dzau is president.

The three Academies work together as the **National Academies of Sciences, Engineering, and Medicine** to provide independent, objective analysis and advice to the nation and conduct other activities to solve complex problems and inform public policy decisions. The National Academies also encourage education and research, recognize outstanding contributions to knowledge, and increase public understanding in matters of science, engineering, and medicine.

Learn more about the National Academies of Sciences, Engineering, and Medicine at **www.nationalacademies.org**.

PLANNING COMMITTEE ON EXPLORING EARLY CHILDHOOD CARE AND EDUCATION LEVERS TO IMPROVE POPULATION HEALTH[1]

MORTON SWARTZ (*Chair*), Chief, Jackson Firm of Medical Service and Infectious Disease Unit, Massachusetts General Hospital
DEBBIE I. CHANG, Senior Vice President, Policy and Prevention, Nemours
MARQUITA F. DAVIS, Deputy Director, Early Childhood Learning, Bill & Melinda Gates Foundation
JENNIFER FREY, Assistant Professor, Graduate School of Education and Human Development, The George Washington University
JACQUELINE JONES, President and Chief Executive Officer, Foundation for Child Development
PAULA M. LANTZ, Professor and Associate Dean for Research and Public Policy, Gerald R. Ford School of Public Policy, University of Michigan
PHYLLIS MEADOWS, Senior Fellow, Health Program, The Kresge Foundation
LARRY PASTI, Senior Director, Big Picture Approach Consulting, Forum for Youth Investment
VALORA WASHINGTON, Chief Executive Officer, Council for Professional Recognition

[1] The National Academies of Sciences, Engineering, and Medicine's planning committees are solely responsible for organizing the workshop, identifying topics, and choosing speakers. The responsibility for the published Proceedings of a Workshop rests with the workshop rapporteur and the institution.

ROUNDTABLE ON POPULATION HEALTH IMPROVEMENT[1]

GEORGE J. ISHAM (*Co-Chair*), Senior Advisor, HealthPartners; Senior Fellow, HealthPartners Institute for Education and Research
SANNE MAGNAN (*Co-Chair*), Adjunct Assistant Professor, University of Minnesota
PHILIP M. ALBERTI, Senior Director, Health Equity Research and Policy, Association of American Medical Colleges
TERRY ALLAN, Health Commissioner, Cuyahoga County Board of Health
JOHN AUERBACH, Executive Director, Trust for America's Health
CATHY BAASE, Chair, Board of Directors, Michigan Health Improvement Alliance, Consultant for Health Strategy, The Dow Chemical Company
DEBBIE I. CHANG, Senior Vice President, Policy and Prevention, Nemours
CHARLES J. FAZIO, Senior Vice President and Medical Director, HealthPartners
GEORGE R. FLORES, Senior Program Officer, The California Endowment
KATHY GERWIG, Vice President, Employee Safety, Health, and Wellness, and Environmental Stewardship Officer, Kaiser Permanente
ALAN GILBERT, Director of Global Government and NGO Strategies, GE Healthymagination
MARY LOU GOEKE, Executive Director, United Way of Santa Cruz County
MARTHE GOLD, Senior Scholar in Residence, The New York Academy of Medicine
MARC N. GOUREVITCH, Professor and Chair, Department of Population Health; Professor, Department of Medicine; Professor, Department of Psychiatry, New York University School of Medicine
GARTH GRAHAM, President, Aetna Foundation
GARY R. GUNDERSON, Vice President, Faith Health, Wake Forest University
WAYNE JONAS, Executive Director, H&S Ventures
ROBERT M. KAPLAN, Professor, Stanford University
DAVID A. KINDIG, Professor Emeritus of Population Health Sciences; Emeritus Vice Chancellor for Health Sciences, University of Wisconsin–Madison

[1] The National Academies of Sciences, Engineering, and Medicine's forums and roundtables do not issue, review, or approve individual documents. The responsibility for the published Proceedings of a Workshop rests with the workshop rapporteur and the institution.

PAULA M. LANTZ, Professor and Associate Dean for Research and Public Policy, Gerald R. Ford School of Public Policy, University of Michigan
MICHELLE LARKIN, Associate Vice President, Associate Chief of Staff, Robert Wood Johnson Foundation
THOMAS A. LaVEIST, Professor and Chair, Department of Health Policy, Milken Institute School of Public Health, The George Washington University
JEFFREY LEVI, Professor, Milken Institute School of Public Health, The George Washington University
SHARRIE McINTOSH, Vice President for Programs, New York State Health Foundation
ROBERT McLELLAN, Chief, Section of Occupational and Environmental Medicine; Medical Director, Live Well/Work Well; Professor, Medicine, Community and Family Medicine and Dartmouth Geisel School of Medicine, Dartmouth-Hitchcock Medical Center
PHYLLIS D. MEADOWS, Senior Fellow, Health Program, The Kresge Foundation
BOBBY MILSTEIN, Director, ReThink Health
JOSÉ T. MONTERO, Director, Office for State, Tribal, Local and Territorial Support; Deputy Director, Centers for Disease Control and Prevention
MARY PITTMAN, President and Chief Executive Officer, Public Health Institute
PAMELA RUSSO, Senior Program Officer, Robert Wood Johnson Foundation

Health and Medicine Division Staff

ALINA BACIU, Study Director
KIMANI HAMILTON-WRAY, Senior Program Assistant
DARLA THOMPSON, Program Officer (*until August 2017*)
ROSE MARIE MARTINEZ, Senior Board Director, Board on Population Health and Public Health Practice

Reviewers

This Proceedings of a Workshop was reviewed in draft form by individuals chosen for their diverse perspectives and technical expertise. The purpose of this independent review is to provide candid and critical comments that will assist the National Academies of Sciences, Engineering, and Medicine in making each published proceedings as sound as possible and to ensure that it meets the institutional standards for quality, objectivity, evidence, and responsiveness to the charge. The review comments and draft manuscript remain confidential to protect the integrity of the process.

We thank the following individuals for their review of this proceedings:

JENNIFER R. FREY, The George Washington University
ELIZABETH GROGINSKY, Government of the District of Columbia
CODY KORNACK, National Head Start Association
ALAN L. MENDELSOHN, New York University School of Medicine
MYETA MOON, United Way Worldwide

Although the reviewers listed above provided many constructive comments and suggestions, they were not asked to endorse the content of the proceedings, nor did they see the final draft before its release. The review of this proceedings was overseen by **HUGH TILSON,** University of North Carolina at Chapel Hill. He was responsible for making certain that an independent examination of this proceedings was carried out in accordance with standards of the National Academies and that all review comments were carefully considered. Responsibility for the final content rests entirely with the rapporteur and the National Academies.

Contents

Acronyms and Abbreviations

CCSSO	Council of Chief State School Officers
CDC	Centers for Disease Control and Prevention
DOHMH	Department of Health and Mental Hygiene (New York City)
ECELC	Early Care & Education Learning Collaborative
EPIC	Executives Partnering to Invest in Children
ESSA	Every Student Succeeds Act
IOM	Institute of Medicine
MTSS	multi-tiered support system
NRC	National Research Council
OACAC	Ozarks Area Community Action Corporation
PBIS	positive behavioral interventions and supports
SEL	social-emotional learning
WIC	Supplemental Nutrition Program for Women, Infants, and Children

1

Introduction[1]

On September 14, 2017, the Roundtable on Population Health Improvement of the National Academies of Sciences, Engineering, and Medicine convened a workshop to explore the intersection of health and early childhood care and education, two key social determinants (or influencing factors) of health. The workshop was held at New York University (NYU) Langone Health in New York City. This workshop follows a 2014 roundtable workshop that considered the interface between the education and health sectors broadly, from research and metrics to cross-sectoral partnerships and financing (IOM, 2015). The 2017 workshop continued that discussion, with a deeper focus on early childhood (birth through age 5) as a critical period in human development and an important opportunity for educational and related interventions. In addition to the 2015 publication, workshop background materials provided to all participants included the report *Transforming the Workforce for Children Birth Through Age 8: A Unifying Foundation* (IOM and NRC, 2015) and other resources to help orient participants to contextual data relevant to this topic.

[1] This workshop was organized by an independent planning committee whose role was limited to identification of topics and speakers. This Proceedings of a Workshop was prepared by the rapporteur as a factual summary of the presentations and discussions that took place at the workshop. Statements, recommendations, and opinions expressed are those of individual presenters and participants and are not necessarily endorsed or verified by the National Academies of Sciences, Engineering, and Medicine; the Health and Medicine Division; or the roundtable, and they should not be construed as reflecting any group consensus.

FOCUSING ON CHILDREN

There are a variety of reasons to focus on early childhood care and education as a population health[2] strategy, said Debbie Chang, the senior vice president of policy and prevention at Nemours Children's Health System (Nemours). Early care and education programs provide an opportunity to connect with families on a routine basis to provide information and support. Sixty percent of children from birth to 5 years, Chang said, spend at least a part of every day in out-of-home settings or under non-parental care while their parents or primary caregivers are working, attending school, participating in job training, or tending to other activities. Families trust their early care and education providers as a source of information and support on child development, health, and parenting. Families see their early care providers nearly every day, and most children spend a great deal of time in early care and education settings. Children learn healthy behaviors early, and early care and education providers are key partners in that learning, Chang said. She referred participants to the work of the Nobel laureate James Heckman and colleagues, who found that children in early childhood programs that included education as well as health and nutrition interventions had improved health outcomes in adulthood, including lower levels of hypertension, metabolic syndrome, and obesity in their 30s (Campbell et al., 2014).

Early care and education programs can promote healthy behaviors through practice change (e.g., creating healthier environments, training care providers to incorporate healthy activities into daily routines and curricula) and policy change. The potential for spread and scale of changes in early care and education practices and policies is great Chang said. By weaving health promotion, preventive care, health literacy, and health care coordination into early care and education environments and making it easier for both health care providers and early care and education providers to coordinate and cooperate through policy levers, we can change the health status of entire geographies of children, Chang said.

WORKSHOP OBJECTIVES

As one of its major activities, the Roundtable on Population Health Improvement sponsors workshops for its members, stakeholders, and the public to discuss issues of importance for improving the nation's health,

[2] Kindig and Stoddart (2003) defined population health as "the health outcomes of a group of individuals, including the distribution of such outcomes within the group" and Jacobson and Teutsch (2012) proposed the term "total population health" to better acknowledge the geopolitical context to population health, its measurement, and policies, including resource allocation, that pertain to it.

said George Isham, a senior advisor at HealthPartners, a senior fellow at the HealthPartners Institute for Education and Research, and a co-chair of the roundtable. The roundtable's vision is of a strong, healthful, and productive society, which cultivates human capital and equal opportunity. This vision rests on the recognition that outcomes such as improved life expectancy, quality of life, and health for all are shaped by interdependent social, economic, environmental, genetic, behavioral, and health care factors, and will require robust national and community-based policies and dependable resources to achieve.

The agenda for this workshop was developed by an independent planning committee that included Debbie Chang, Marquita Davis, Jennifer Frey, Jacqueline Jones, Paula Lantz, Phyllis Meadows, Larry Pasti, Morton Swartz, and Valora Washington. (The planning committee's Statement of Task is provided in Box 1-1.) The workshop was designed to explore the intersection of health and early care and education (birth through age 5), with particular attention paid to equity,[3] and across all early care and education settings. The workshop agenda was developed by the planning committee to meet the following objectives:

- Highlight what is working at the intersection of health and early care and education; discuss the importance of early care and education in achieving overall goals for early childhood development; and consider current priorities.
- Provide examples of successful initiatives focused on early care and education and health.
- Create space for conversations around the examples provided, including spread and scale for greater impact, sustainability (including funding models), the collection of relevant data, and the identification of gaps that need to be addressed.

ORGANIZATION OF THE WORKSHOP AND PROCEEDINGS

This proceedings summarizes the presentations and discussions that took place at the workshop Exploring Early Childhood Care and Education Levers to Improve Population Health. The workshop was organized around three panel sessions consisting of presentations and panel

[3] See, for example, the definition of "health equity" in a 2017 National Academies report, a definition that could similarly be applied to equity in an early childhood education context. "Health equity is the state in which everyone has the opportunity to attain full health potential and no one is disadvantaged from achieving this potential because of social position or any other socially defined circumstance. In this report promoting health equity means creating the conditions where individuals and communities have what they need to enjoy full, healthy lives" (NASEM, 2017, p. 32).

BOX 1-1
Planning Committee Statement of Task

An ad hoc committee will plan and convene a 1-day public workshop that will build on the June 2014 workshop hosted by the Roundtable on Population Health Improvement, again featuring invited presentations and discussion on research, policy, and practice at the intersection of health and education, this time with a narrower focus on the early childhood period. The committee will develop the agenda and identify meeting objectives, select appropriate speakers, and moderate the discussions. The workshop will include the perspectives of experts from the health, education, and other relevant sectors and may explore such topics as the state of the evidence, shared outcomes/metrics, early childhood education financing, and ways that health sector leaders can partner with and support education sector counterparts. Proceedings based on the presentations and discussions at the workshop will be prepared by a designated rapporteur in accordance with institutional guidelines.

discussions. Each panel session was followed by a "gallery walk" that gave participants the opportunity to reflect on the panel discussion with other attendees and respond (in writing) to specific questions that were posed on posters in a meeting room adjacent to the auditorium where the workshop took place. Upon reconvening in plenary session, the session moderators reported and summarized individual participants' comments from the gallery walk.

The first panel explored some aspects of the evidence available at the intersection of health with early care and education, including examples of what works in practice and at the policy level to influence children's health and development/educational outcomes (Chapter 2). The second panel shared lessons learned from cross-sector collaborations in the health and early care and education sectors (Chapter 3). The final panel focused on policy challenges and opportunities, including issues related to financing, the workforce, and equity (Chapter 4). The workshop concluded with summary remarks and reflections on the discussions by Isham and Meadows (Chapter 5). The appendixes to the proceedings include an overview of the input shared in individual participant comments during the gallery walk interactive portions of the workshop and a compendium of links and citations pertaining to the many programs described or mentioned by the day's presenters.

2

Exploring the Evidence at the Intersection of Early Care and Education with Health

The first panel discussed the importance of early care and education in achieving overall goals for early childhood development, and it explored the evidence concerning effective programs at the intersection of health and early care and education. The opening presentation was given by Judith Carta, the director of the Bridging the Word Gap Research Network, interim director of Juniper Gardens Children's Project, a senior scientist at the Institute for Lifespan Studies, and a professor of special education at the University of Kansas. Carta described several examples of multi-sector collaboration on early language promotion and closing the word gap. Laurie Brotman, the Bezos Family Foundation Professor of Early Childhood Development in the Department of Population Health at New York University (NYU), discussed family-centered early childhood education as a lever to improve population health and promote health equity. Allison Gertel-Rosenberg, the director of National Prevention and Practice at Nemours, described a collaborative model to bring early care providers together to learn how to change their policies and practices related to healthy eating and physical activity. She also discussed the spread and scale of that collaborative model into a national collaborative. In a joint presentation, Jodie Whiteman, the director of professional development at Zero to Three, and Sarah LeMoine, the director of early childhood workforce innovations at Zero to Three, discussed several examples of professional development programs at the intersection of the health sector and the early care and education sector, including cross-sector core competencies for those working with children prenatal through age 5 and critical competencies for infant/toddler educators. The session was moderated by Danielle Ewen, a senior policy advisor at EducationCounsel, LLC.

Following the presentations and discussion, participants moved to the adjacent gallery to reflect on the panel discussion with other attendees, and to consider specific questions that were posed on posters around the gallery. Upon reconvening in plenary session, Valora Washington, the chief executive officer of the Council for Professional Recognition, moderated a discussion of the responses to the questions. (Session highlights are presented in Box 2-1.)

BOX 2-1
Highlights and Main Points Made by Individual Speakers[a]

- Closing the word gap through prevention (e.g., community-wide public awareness, training, and tools for new parents) and intervention (evidence-based language development strategies) promotes resilience, reduces disparities, and gives children a stronger language background, which will influence multiple outcomes in their lives (e.g., academic, social and emotional, health). Current multi-sector work is often occurring in parallel, and true collaboration and integration across sectors are needed. (Carta)
- Evidence-based programs that create safe, nurturing, and predictable environments for children can lead to positive child outcomes in terms of self-regulation, academic achievement, and mental and physical health. Moving from efficacy data and the promise of early interventions to actually implementing, evaluating, and improv ing at scale depends on relationships, partnerships, and trust. (Brotman)
- Be responsive to the needs of local partners, who know their community best; use creative incentives to foster engagement; and think about sustainability and integration into existing systems at every point. (Gertel-Rosenberg)
- Caring for infants and toddlers requires a holistic approach, and specialized competencies can positively affect the daily interactions that educators have with very young children, ages 0 to 3. (LeMoine, Whiteman)
- Early childhood care and education can be a lever to promote health equity. Attention to equity in policies, practices, and programs is important for improving childhood outcomes. (Brotman, LeMoine)

[a] This list is the rapporteur's summary of the main points made by individual speakers and participants (noted in parentheses) and does not reflect any consensus among workshop participants or endorsement by the National Academies of Sciences, Engineering, and Medicine.

CLOSING THE WORD GAP[1]

By age 3, a low-income child has typically heard 30 million fewer words than a child from an upper income background (Hart and Risley, 1995). This is known as the *word gap*, Carta said. Early language exposure has important consequences for vocabulary development, literacy, school success, and life outcomes. Vocabulary by age 3 is an important predictor of reading by third grade, Carta continued, and at age 3 children from higher-income homes have double the vocabulary of those from lower-income homes. Reading in third grade is a critical predictor for later life success and is the most important predictor of high school graduation. Children who cannot read in third grade are four times more likely to drop out of high school and six times more likely to drop out of high school if they are also living in poverty. This discrepancy in language experience between higher- and lower-income children has been known for a long time, Carta said, and it is essentially a health disparity and a life outcome disparity.

There are evidence-based interventions for promoting language in infants and toddlers, including simple behaviors that parents and caregivers can embed in their daily routines to provide a rich language experience to children. The tools for reducing the word gap are available, Carta said, but the importance of talking with young children even before they can speak is not widely known. Closing the word gap will require both prevention and intervention, Carta said. Prevention includes fostering a broader public awareness of the importance of talking to young children and providing a greater variety of programs with training and advice for parents and early educators on ways to promote language. Intervention involves the use of evidence-based strategies that can change how parents, caregivers, and early educators interact with children to promote language.

Bridging the Word Gap Research Network

The Bridging the Word Gap Research Network[2] was funded by the Health Resources and Services Administration in 2014 to bring together agencies and individuals across sectors who are already working to address the word gap. The goal of the network is to reduce the vocabulary gap of children from lower-income backgrounds by increasing their

[1] This section is the rapporteur's synopsis of the presentation by Judith Carta, and the statements are not endorsed or verified by the National Academies of Sciences, Engineering, and Medicine.

[2] For more information, see http://www.bwgresnet.res.ku.edu (accessed October 30, 2017).

language learning experiences. The network, Carta explained, is synthesizing the research around prevention and intervention to identify what works to promote children's language and is sharing the most effective practices with stakeholders across disciplines that can have an impact on children's language development. The network is also identifying research gaps and developing new studies and innovations for prevention and intervention. In this regard, the network has launched a practice-based research collaborative, which Carta described as a partnership among "hotspots of innovation." Carta shared several examples of projects from the collaborative.

Community-Wide Public Awareness

Bringing together multiple agencies and multiple sectors in a community is one way of getting the word out, Carta said. One example of this approach is Too Small to Fail, a joint initiative of the Clinton Foundation and the Opportunity Institute. This public awareness campaign is working with communities to promote recognition of the importance of early brain and language development. The campaign engages community leaders across multiple sectors (e.g., pediatricians, housing, early education, faith-based organizations, community-based organizations, businesses, and others) to provide parents with tools that will help them talk, read, and sing with their young children. The goal, Carta stated, is to get the message out in the places where families go (e.g., laundromats, supermarkets, playgrounds) and to give parents ideas for what they can talk about with their children wherever they spend time together.

Another example provided by Carta is City's First Readers, an initiative of the New York City Council, which is a multi-sector collaboration fostering early language and literacy through parent engagement workshops, reading opportunities, book distribution, and other activities. The initiative brings together a diverse array of programs from a number of sectors, such as libraries; pediatric settings; the United Way; early childhood education organizations; community-based, literacy-promoting organizations; and home-visiting organizations.

Population-Based Interventions in Pediatric Settings

Another strategy for population-based language interventions, Carta said, is to engage sectors that interact with high numbers of families of young children, such as the pediatric public health sector. Talk With Me Baby is Georgia's public health sector intervention to bridge the word gap. This public action campaign engages pediatric providers and nutritionists to spread the message that parents are providing "language nutrition" for their children when they interact and talk with them. Just as children need an adequate amount of food to grow and thrive, so they also need language, Carta said. When parents bring their child for well visits, the providers coach them on age-appropriate activities to promote language development. This initiative is reaching almost all lower-income children within the state of Georgia, she said.

Reach Out and Read is a national program aimed at making literacy a standard part of pediatric primary care. The program has a broad reach and is evidence based, with more than 15 studies supporting its effectiveness. Reach Out and Read is currently reaching 4.5 million children per year, or more than 25 percent of all low-income children ages 6 months to 5 years in the United States, Carta said. At $25 per child per year, this is an example of a low-cost initiative that is being successfully scaled.

Individual Interventions Teaching Parents Language-Promoting Strategies

The final area of intervention discussed by Carta was evidence-based approaches that provide parents with specific training in language-promoting strategies they can use with their children. She described three examples: the Video Interaction Project (which also takes place at pediatric health care visits), which promotes parent–child interaction through one-on-one support; Thirty Million Words, which informs parents about the importance of language and literacy shortly after a child's birth while they are still in the hospital and then has a home visit to teach simple strategies when the child reaches 6 months; and Tools for Advancing Language in Kids, which is a professional development program for early childhood educators.

Potential Challenges for Future Work

In summary, Carta concluded, multi-sector collaboration to close the word gap is already taking place. Sectors are working together on public awareness campaigns in communities, and agencies are working together across sectors toward the common goals of promoting language and early literacy. Carta noted, however, that multi-sector work is often occurring in parallel—that is, with the various entities working side by side on similar goals—and there is still room to grow in terms of true collaboration and integration across sectors. Such collaboration and integration would include, for example, the sharing of data across sectors and more early screening in pediatric settings, with referrals to more intensive services in early childhood education or home-visiting programs.

Carta noted that through multi-sector collaboration, word gap interventions can be developed and deployed that can strengthen parental bonds, promote resilience, and give children a stronger language background, which will influence multiple outcomes in their lives (e.g., academic achievement, social and emotional development, health outcomes). Prevention and intervention to address the word gap can help ensure that all children enter kindergarten on track, which will support better health and educational outcomes in the long term.

A participant asked a question about the types of interventions available to support language development in children with hearing impairments. Carta said that the implications of the word gap for children who are hearing impaired are similar to those for children who can hear. She referred participants to the work of Dana Suskind at The University of Chicago. Suskind's interest in early language experience emerged after learning that among hearing impaired children who had received cochlear implants, language development in children from higher-income areas in Chicago progressed well, but children from the lower-income areas continued to show considerable delay in their language development.

FAMILY-CENTERED EARLY CHILDHOOD EDUCATION[3]

Poverty, adverse childhood experiences, and racism affect all aspects of child development, Brotman said, including behavioral, physical, cognitive, social, and emotional development. There are many different mechanisms through which poverty and adversity influence these outcomes, she said, but a key mechanism is through the development of self-regulation. During the preschool period, self-regulation skills begin to come together as children hone their ability to pay attention, control impulses, delay gratification, and regulate their emotions, Brotman explained, and these skills are malleable early on. With this evidence in mind, ParentCorps was developed by NYU Langone Health as an enhancement to pre-K programs that supports leaders, teachers, and parents in creating safe, nurturing, and predictable environments for children.[4]

ParentCorps

The goal of ParentCorps, Brotman said, is to promote population health and reduce socioeconomic disparities through a family-centered intervention that is broadly available, engaging, and effective for low-

[3] This section is the rapporteur's synopsis of the presentation by Laurie Brotman, and the statements are not endorsed or verified by the National Academies of Sciences, Engineering, and Medicine.

[4] For more information, see https://med.nyu.edu/pophealth/divisions/cehd/parentcorps (accessed October 30, 2017).

income, culturally diverse families. The program is built on five principles, each based on decades of research and rooted in studies in clinical and developmental psychology. First, ParentCorps was designed to be a universal enhancement to pre-K, in order to achieve maximum reach and acceptability. Second, the program was designed to be embedded in schools and facilitated by school staff, which would foster cost efficiencies and sustainability by building on existing structure and capabilities. Third, the program is timed with the transition to school, at the time when child self-regulation is developing and parents are open to change and motivated to be involved in supporting their children's learning. Fourth, ParentCorps has multiple components to support the home and classroom environment and also family engagement. Finally, at the core of ParentCorps is a group-based parenting program that places culture at the center in order to build social capital and create a network of empowered parents.

The three main components of ParentCorps are schools, classrooms, and homes, Brotman said. The program influences the school environment through professional learning for leaders, pre-K teachers, mental health professionals in the schools, and family support staff. The home environment is influenced through a 14-session parenting program, which covers topics from goals, routines, and responsibilities to enjoying mealtime together, the power of play, and effective discipline. The program influences classrooms through a program for pre-K students called Friends School. The 14 lessons of the Friends School curriculum span such topics as making friends and sharing; paying attention; saying "please," "thank you," "sorry," and "excuse me;" identifying feelings (happy, sad, mad, scared); taking care of oneself; and celebrating people's differences. Brotman listed the topics covered during different 2-hour activity sessions, which included free play, the lesson topic, a welcome circle, an activity, physical exercise, food review, calm down techniques, and mealtime with the teacher.

ParentCorps is based on a theory of change that the school, home, and classroom program components come together to create safe, nurturing, and predictable environments; effective family engagement and strong parent–teacher relationships; and social and emotional skills. The result is positive child outcomes in terms of self-regulation, academic achievement, mental health, and physical health (see Figure 2-1).

The theory of change is supported by two decades of evidence from two large randomized controlled trials in New York City in high-poverty schools with pre-K programs, Brotman said. These studies show that this program can lead to short- and long-term changes for children and families. Specifically, replicated evidence shows that the program leads to

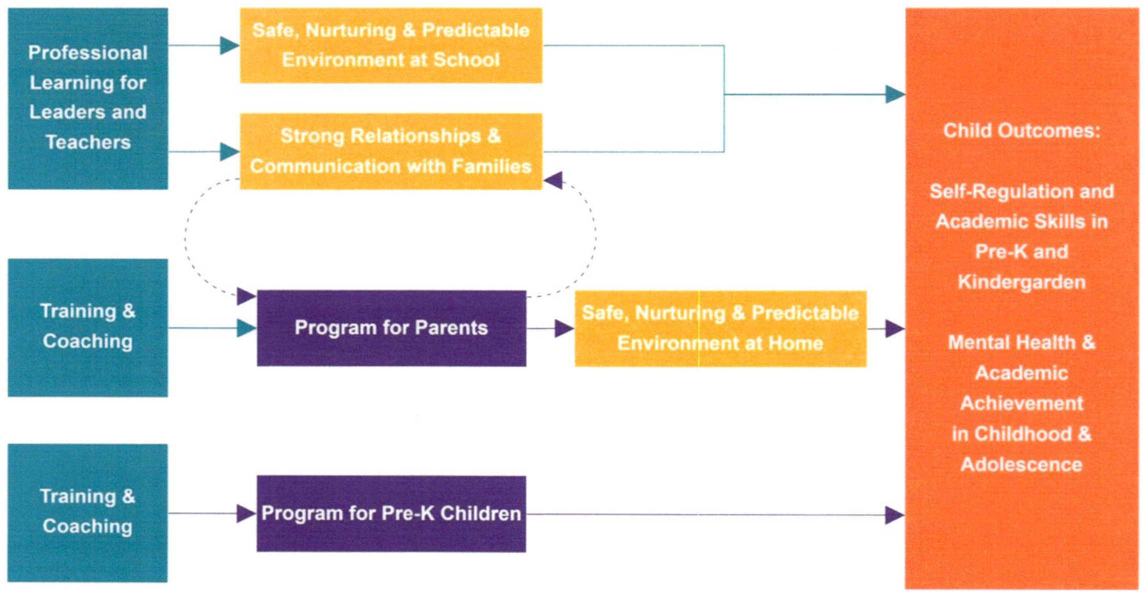

FIGURE 2-1 ParentCorps theory of change.
SOURCE: Brotman presentation, September 14, 2017.

- positive parenting practices that lead to safe, nurturing, and predictable environments at home and parental involvement in learning, both at home and in the classroom;
- positive classroom environments that are safe, nurturing, and predictable as well as strong family engagement;
- increased school readiness, both in terms of self-regulation and pre-academic skills (literacy and math); and
- sustained impact (pre-K through second grade thus far) on academic achievement (test scores, teacher ratings), mental health outcomes (behavioral and emotional), and physical health (obesity/body mass index [BMI], healthy behaviors).

With a successful, evidence-based program in place, the next step was to take ParentCorps to scale in New York City, Brotman said. As of September 2017, ParentCorps was in place in 35 high-poverty schools and centers in five boroughs, with plans for further expansion in 2018, she said. Working with partners in the Department of Education, Brotman said, a three-tiered model for spreading ParentCorps's evidence-based practices to two other initiatives was developed. New York has invested in Pre-K for All, a program to give all children in New York City an opportunity to engage in full-day pre-K, and in NYC Pre-K Thrive, a component of ThriveNYC, a mayoral initiative to support mental health. The ParentCorps program is

1. providing universal supports to all 1,870 Pre-K for All programs, which serve 70,000 children annually;
2. spreading evidence-based practices through intensive professional learning in 350 Pre-K for All programs; and
3. continuing to deliver ParentCorps in 55 Pre-K for All programs.

Furthermore, an evaluation plan has been developed in partnership with the Department of Education; the plan includes three randomized controlled trials to assess implementation and effectiveness and to rigorously evaluate the scale-up initiative.

Potential Opportunities, Challenges, and Future Directions

The opportunities to partner with education providers and leaders to implement health promotion programs are enormous, Brotman concluded. The greatest challenge, she said, will be moving from the efficacy data and the promise of these interventions to actually implementing, evaluating, and improving at scale. Moving forward, Brotman said, will depend on relationships, partnerships, and trust.

LEARNING COLLABORATIVES

Nemours has been working at the intersection of early care and education and health for some time, Gertel-Rosenberg said. The company first worked with partners in the state of Delaware to change regulations affecting early care and education so that they better reflected best practices in healthy eating and physical activity. Those changes affected the 54,000 children in Delaware who were in early care and education settings on a regular basis, she said.

Nemours has also had success at the practice level, establishing a collaborative model that brought early care providers in Delaware together in groups to learn together how to change their policies and practices related to healthy eating and physical activity. Nemours engaged early care providers who were serving about 2,700 children in Delaware. Gertel-Rosenberg said that 100 percent of the providers made changes in either healthy eating or physical activity and that 81 percent of them made changes in both. Nemours found that early care providers were eager for this type of information, including actionable steps—a pattern that continued with the launch of Let's Move! Child Care in 2011. A decision was made to try to spread and scale the early care and education learning collaborative model beyond Delaware.

National Early Care and Education Learning Collaborative

With a 5-year cooperative agreement with the Centers for Disease Control and Prevention (CDC), Nemours was able to leverage and expand the collaborative work that had been successful in Delaware, and in 2012 the national Early Care & Education Learning Collaborative (ECELC) was launched.[5] The ECELC has now been implemented in 10 states (Alabama, Arizona, California, Florida, Indiana, Kansas, Kentucky, Missouri, New Jersey, and Virginia). More than 2,200 early care and education programs serving more than 191,000 children have taken part in 106 collaboratives across the country. Evaluation shows that these providers are making significant changes in practices related to nutrition, physical activity, breastfeeding, screen time, and other areas, Gertel-Rosenberg said.

The ECELC has two main parts. A practice component offers early care providers the tools and technical assistance to change the practices in their care centers or family child care homes. There are best practices for physical activity, screen time, breastfeeding, and other areas. A systems change component helps to foster sustainability. This work is done via state or local plans that are developed by state partners in coordination

[5] For more information, see www.healthykidshealthyfuture.org (accessed October 30, 2017).

with other partners in the state. States and localities are provided with technical assistance and peer support from other states that have gone through similar sustainability and integration opportunities.

Lessons Learned

Gertel-Rosenberg shared four key lessons from the scale-up of the ECELC. Be responsive to the needs of partners and early care and education providers, she said. State and local partners know their geography and their communities, and they can help with uptake in their areas. The curriculum is customizable, and the implementation is reflective of what is needed in the states and communities. For example, the curriculum has been translated into Spanish, and there is now a family child care curriculum. In Arizona the ECELC was aligned with and supported the goals of the state's existing Empower initiative to help children grow up healthy.

Another lesson is that incentives foster engagement. This is not limited to financial incentives, Gertel-Rosenberg said, and she emphasized opportunities to think outside the box. One incentive that brought people to the table, for example, was ensuring that the learning sessions and the action periods in between were eligible for continuing education hours or clock hours.

Leverage the initial investment with additional investment, Gertel-Rosenberg said. Nemours was able to increase the spread of ECELC and provide additional enhancements beyond what was initially funded by CDC by partnering with private foundations to meet shared needs. These partners wanted to have collaboratives in additional places, for example, or they wanted to provide durable goods to help providers implement the best practices (e.g., family-style dining, physical activity), or they wanted to pilot innovations on such topics as parent engagement, centralized kitchens for child care centers, or variations on the implementation of the model. Nemours also worked with the states to determine how their funding could best be leveraged. In Florida, for example, funding from CDC's 1305 program[6] was used to spread the learning collaboratives to additional sites in the state.

Finally, Gertel-Rosenberg advised participants to think about integration and sustainability at the beginning, middle, end, and every point in between. They could consider, for instance, integrating into existing systems, especially other child-serving systems. Each state provides examples of how to integrate and embed the content and demonstrate

[6] State Public Health Actions to Prevent and Control Diabetes, Heart Disease, Obesity and Associated Risk Factors and Promote School Health (DP13-1305). See https://www.cdc.gov/chronicdisease/about/state-public-health-actions.htm (accessed October 30, 2017).

value, she said. In Orange County, Florida, for example, a quality rating and improvement system pilot awards points for healthy eating and physical activity, which creates an additional incentive for early care and education programs to ensure that this content is embedded. A preschool in Jefferson County, Kentucky, highlighted the impact of implementing family-style dining at snack time. They noticed significant changes in food behaviors as well as increased independence that carried over to other activities (e.g., students setting up their own cots or initiating other self-care activities without adult prompts). As the ECELC project has ended in some states, those states have chosen to continue funding the project coordinators and the work.

THE PROVEN POWER OF EARLY CONNECTIONS[7]

Since 1977, LeMoine said, Zero to Three has been translating research on how the youngest children think, learn, and interact with the important adults in their lives into helpful tools, services, and practical resources for parents, policy makers, and professionals.[8] The mission of Zero to Three is to ensure that all babies and toddlers have a strong start in life. Zero to Three envisions a society that has the knowledge and the will to support all infants and toddlers in reaching their full potential. LeMoine emphasized the urgency of that mission, and she shared a quote from the Institute of Medicine and the National Research Council (IOM and NRC) consensus report *Transforming the Workforce for Children Birth Through Age 8: A Unifying Foundation*:

> concerted attention is needed to incorporate . . . the workforce development needs of those who provide care and education for infants and toddlers. These professionals have historically had the weakest, least explicit and coherent, and least resourced infrastructure for professional learning and workforce supports. (IOM and NRC, 2015, p. 504)

Zero to Three: Professional Development Initiatives

Whiteman noted the variety of different professionals who touch the lives of very young children and families. She discussed several examples of the work that Zero to Three is doing at the intersection of the health sector and the early care and education sector, spanning physical health,

[7] This section is the rapporteur's synopsis of the presentation by Sarah LeMoine and Jody Whiteman, and the statements are not endorsed or verified by the National Academies of Sciences, Engineering, and Medicine.

[8] See https://www.zerotothree.org (accessed October 30, 2017).

mental health, child welfare, and social services; early identification and intervention; and early care and education.

One such example, Knowledge and Know-How: Nurturing Child Well-Being, is a program of eight online 1-hour lessons for professionals. Whitman said that the simple theory of change model is based on the integration of cross-sector professionals as well as the integration of health, well-being, mental health, early intervention,[9] and the opportunity to share language. Immediate outcomes include knowledge gains, strengthened parent–provider relationships, and the promotion of cross-sector collaboration. Longer-term outcomes include increased support for families, optimal development for infants and toddlers, and a reduced risk of child maltreatment.

Whiteman also described Cross-Sector Core Competencies for the Prenatal Through Age Five Field, a program funded by First Five LA. This professional development resource covers eight competency areas: early childhood development; family-centered practice; relationship-based practice; health and developmental protective and risk factors; cultural and linguistic responsiveness; leadership; professional and ethical practices; and service planning, coordination, and collaboration. These competencies build on and are aligned with related professional criteria, and they are intended to enhance cross-sector collaboration and foster shared language.

LeMoine described a related example focused on Critical Competencies for Infant-Toddler Educators. This resource builds on the cross-sector collaborative foundation. Caring for infants and toddlers requires a holistic approach, she said, and educators play a key role in supporting and nurturing all aspects of infant/toddler learning and development. In the best-case scenario, LeMoine said, educators partner with families and with other sectors and disciplines to create a comprehensive environment that protects, engages, and nurtures children. In considering its decades of work with numerous partners, Zero to Three identified a persistent gap found in the daily interactions between infants-toddlers and their educators. These educators often receive workforce training geared intentionally toward the pre-K age group and then return to work to care for, say, a 6-month-old, unclear on how to transfer their new knowledge to their very young charges. To address this, Zero to Three developed specialized competencies that include sector-, discipline-, role-, and age-specific skills. In implementing these competencies, Zero to Three is supplementing and building on what already exists in the states. There is training for the pro-

[9] "Early intervention" generally refers to services defined in Part C of the Individuals with Disabilities Education and Improvement Act (IDEA). For more information, see http://idea.ed.gov/part-c/search/new.html (accessed January 23, 2018).

fessional development providers who train early care educators as well as support and training for the educators themselves to reflect on and positively impact their daily practices with infants and toddlers. LeMoine said that Zero to Three applies a diversity, fairness, and equity lens to each of the practices that are included in the critical competencies, not only because educators work with a diverse population but also because educators themselves are diverse. The critical competencies also address working with vulnerable populations and multi-language learners.

Sometimes children need more than what even the most skilled educator can provide, LeMoine said, and Zero to Three also emphasizes a multi-disciplinary approach to help educators connect with families in meaningful ways and understand where their role might end and where other partners and support services can step in (e.g., identification of children who may need additional specialized services, coordination with medical partners, referring for mental health evaluation).

DISCUSSION

To start the discussion, Ewen listed some of the topics raised in the presentations, including specific health and development issues such as vocabulary gaps, nutrition, executive function,[10] and self-regulation; the importance of taking equity into account; and the need to engage and share information with the many diverse stakeholders involved in some way in children's health, including parents and caregivers, pediatricians, mental health providers, community service providers, social service providers, and others. Speakers also emphasized the importance of cross-sector collaboration and partnerships; the integration of programs and services to foster sustainability; and evidence to support spread and scale of programs. The discussion centered on metrics and measurements—in particular, on assessing the impact of programs on equity and on metrics of mental and physical health outcomes in young children.

Assessing Equity

Phillip Alberti of the Association of American Medical Colleges acknowledged the attention to equity in the programs discussed and

[10] Harvard University's Center on the Developing Child provides the following definition: "Executive function and self-regulation skills are the mental processes that enable us to plan, focus attention, remember instructions, and juggle multiple tasks successfully. Just as an air traffic control system at a busy airport safely manages the arrivals and departures of many aircraft on multiple runways, the brain needs this skill set to filter distractions, prioritize tasks, set and achieve goals, and control impulses," see https://developingchild.harvard.edu/science/key-concepts/executive-function (accessed January 22, 2018).

asked whether disparities-focused metrics or equity-sensitive metrics were assessed in order to understand how the programs were affecting the gaps. He raised the need for implementation science, noting that one size will not fit all in every program, school, or community, and he asked whether anyone was studying the types of adaptations that might be needed to ensure that all communities benefit equally.

LeMoine responded that the Harris Foundation's Infant Mental Health Tenets, which are diversity informed, were applied as overarching principles in developing Zero to Three's critical competencies. There are also measures tied into state systems that are used to assess how well diversity, fairness, and equity are being applied in each of the competency areas. Reflection tools tied to specific competency areas are used at the individual practice level. At the systems level, Zero to Three is conducting pilot studies with data fields. There is also attention to implementation science, LeMoine said. For example, teams are required to come together for direct service training. This is a significant commitment, she added, and there is a readiness-for-change component to the program, where the teams reflect beforehand.

Brotman reiterated that ParentCorps is focused both on promoting population health and on reducing disparities. Since its inception, the program has been careful to look at how it affects different subgroups, paying attention to gender, race/ethnicity, and children who come to pre-K with low self-regulation skills. ParentCorps has also been deeply engaged in racial equity work at all levels and is working with the Pacific Education Group consulting firm, Brotman added. There is a tremendous amount of work to do, she said, in order to understand what it means to apply a racial equity lens to all of the components of a program (e.g., the population as well as workforce diversity, including diversity of the implementation team, coaches, trainers, researchers) and to tie that together with prevention science, developmental science, implementation science, and improvement science.

Measuring Mental and Physical Health Outcomes

Aly Richards of the Permanent Fund for Vermont's Children noted the challenges of identifying the right metrics to use for child mental health and physical health outcomes, especially metrics that translate to health and mental health partners. She asked specifically about the teacher ratings used by ParentCorps and also about whether ParentCorps has been able to leverage those metrics and outcomes to secure funding. Brotman replied that the randomized controlled trials of the ParentCorps model used the Behavior Assessment System for Children, which includes teacher ratings and parent ratings. Moving forward, ParentCorps is working in partnership with the Department of Education on existing assessments for quality and outcomes. The quality discussion is somewhat easier to have, she said, even though the topic is complicated. Discussions about measuring children's behavior and mental health face numerous complexities. In New York City there is systematic, annual measurement of BMI, and ways to measure academic outcomes in school-age children, but there is no systematic way yet to measure mental health outcomes.

Terry Allan of the Cuyahoga County Health Department in greater Cleveland asked about the durability over time of health outcomes associated with the ParentCorps program. Brotman responded that there are replicated findings from one study that followed children through early adolescence and from another that has thus far followed the children through second grade. In the latter, the children will continue to be followed as they transition to middle school, while those in the earliest cohorts will be followed as they transition to high school. There are very clear patterns of separation, very early on in pre-K, Brotman said, as the children without intervention escalate on the obesity scale, and that separation continues to grow over time.

GALLERY WALK REFLECTIONS

Following the panel discussion, participants moved to the gallery to consider the following questions:

- How can the field better apply what is known at the interface of early care and education and health (e.g., screening for developmental milestones)?
- What are the gaps that need to be prioritized?
- What new insights can be offered?

Upon reconvening, Washington summarized individual participants' responses to the questions posed in the gallery and moderated the discussion. Health outcomes are among the most well-documented benefits of programs that serve young children, Washington said, and she emphasized the need to consider how best to leverage this fact. She observed that there were many diverse comments shared by individual participants during the gallery walk, and she framed the comments in terms of four principles:

- **Respect.** Many of the individual comments focused on how best to respect families in this work and on the importance of asking parents what they want.
- **Competence.** There were many comments concerning how this work will actually be done. Questions were posted regarding infra-

structure, how sectors work together, and whether there is a common language that enables communication across these sectors, for example.

- **Strengths.** Participant comments also raised the issue of how best to build on the current knowledge base and not "reinvent the wheel." This work has been going on for a long time, Washington said, and participants highlighted the need to build upon existing strengths and leverage the prior work. Questions were raised about the need for public campaigns to advertise and promote these strengths.
- **Equity.** Washington noted that there were only a few comments posted about equity, and she prompted participants to consider the issue further, including where equity ranks in the work on the intersection between early childhood care and health.

Prevention of Disparities: Spreading and Scaling Programs That Work

In considering gaps to be prioritized, Alan Mendelsohn of NYU suggested that greater focus is needed on the role that the health care system can play in the prevention of disparities in early child development and school readiness. He referred to the examples provided by Carta and other panelists and emphasized the importance of this role of the health care system as a focus, rather than an afterthought, in policy conversations. He observed that the pediatric platform is quite good at screening and identifying families with emergent problems (e.g., parent–child challenges; developmental statuses that require referral for early intervention or other services). He suggested that a prime opportunity to engage families during the critical birth to age 3 period is during the many pediatric primary care visits that occur during this time frame (at least seven in the first year of life). Parents come with an interest in knowing about their children's development and behavior. The Reach Out and Read program, which incorporates books into pediatric care (discussed by Carta), is an example of working to prevent child development disparities before they occur, he said. These programs have been shown to be effective, and some, he added, are being effectively scaled (as discussed by Carta, Reach Out and Read is currently reaching more than 25 percent of low-income children in the United States from age 6 months to 5 years).

Isham said it would be important to understand what factors or characteristics of the Reach Out and Read program led to the broad reach that it has achieved thus far. Understanding how such programs are spread will also be important to efforts to reduce disparity, he added. For example, if a program is covered or incentivized by insurance, that would limit spread to the population that has the relevant insurance coverage.

Alan Mendelsohn said that one reason it is possible to reach that 25 percent of low-income families through health care is because many are covered by Medicaid and come in for the many early childhood pediatric visits for vaccines, screenings, and other services. With regard to dissemination and implementation across practices, he referred participants to the work of Perri Klass and his colleagues at NYU (for example, see Klass et al., 2009). The model includes, for example, grassroots efforts, making literacy promotion part of the pediatric training in residency programs, and developing regional organizations and infrastructure to allow for central and local support for the implementation of the program.

Whiteman said that Zero to Three is the home of Healthy Steps, a program that trains and houses Healthy Steps specialists in pediatric offices to work with families on all aspects of behavioral health. Zero to Three is now working on taking this program to scale. Whiteman noted that Zero to Three is currently advocating at the federal and state policy levels and working with health maintenance organizations and Medicaid to address reimbursement issues for these services. For example, billing and reimbursement may depend on the specific license a Healthy Steps specialist has.

Bonnie Kerker of the NYU Department of Population Health agreed with Mendelsohn and said that it will be critical to expand the focus of the pediatric visit to include, in addition to developmental programs, mental health and social aspects of the family environment. These areas also have tremendous impact on both immediate and longer-term outcomes for children and thus need greater attention. She also suggested that there is a need to start before the pediatrics office—in the obstetrician/gynecologists office—as data show that in order to ensure positive outcomes for children, social, emotional, and other aspects of child health need to be addressed even before a woman becomes pregnant.

Washington noted that prevention is often tied to funding (i.e., funding decisions based on whether prevention is done). Larry Pasti of the Forum for Youth Investment said that many family insurance plans now incentivize prevention for adults—for example, by offering discounts on gym memberships or other incentives—but such incentives have not yet benefited children or infants. He suggested that insurance companies help fund preventive initiatives that can have long-term health benefits for children, such as the types of reading programs discussed.

Funding, Financing, and Reimbursement

Paula Lantz of the Gerald R. Ford School of Public Policy at the University of Michigan suggested that there is a need to add funding and financing to the principles listed by Washington. It is important to include a cost component in evaluations in order to better understand both the costs and the value of interventions and to demonstrate the costs and value to policy makers and other funders. She also spoke of the need to consider different funding models, especially as they relate to different kinds of communities. For example, how can high-quality pre-K be funded so that inequities will not become reinforced and widened? Washington agreed that the issue of funding is applicable to all of the principles she listed.

A participant pointed to the ongoing struggle between reimbursement methodology and the movement toward value-based payment. In New York, for example, there are more than 2 million children in managed care, which is rapidly transitioning to value-based payment models. New York State recently released a value-based payment model for pediatrics that is focused on achieving population health–level impacts. The model addresses the need to transition to yet-to-be-developed common metrics between the early education sector and pediatrics. These are ambitious measures, she added. She urged the National Academies to elevate the conversation about expanding quality measures from not just whether a well-child visit is done, to whether that well-child visit includes a population health primary prevention focus and whether it could eventually align goals with early care and education.

3

Cross-Sector Collaboration

Research has shown that the foundations of health are built in the earliest years, said session moderator Debbie Chang of Nemours. Young children are particularly sensitive to the social determinants of health. Those social determinants exist in multiple sectors, including housing, early care and education, school-age education, business, and health care, among others. In this session, the panelists discussed collaboration among the various sectors at the intersection of early care and education and health. George Askew, the deputy commissioner of the Division of Family and Child Health in the New York City Department of Health and Mental Hygiene (DOHMH), provided examples of cross-sector initiatives concerning early care and education and health across the agency. Kimberly Shinn-Brown, the program director of the Ozarks Area Community Action Corporation (OACAC) Head Start program in Springfield, Missouri, shared examples of how Head Start can improve population health and health equity for children. Krista Scott, the senior director of Health Policy at Child Care Aware, described how state child care agencies are working to make care settings healthier through professional development, settings standards, and investing in quality. Michelle Suarez, an early childhood developer with Prosper Lincoln at Nebraska Children and Families Foundation, described the development of a cross-sector community agenda to improve the health and prosperity of Lincoln, targeting early childhood for health, wellness, and prevention interventions.

Following the presentations and discussion, participants moved to the adjacent gallery to reflect on the panel discussion with other attendees and to consider specific questions that were posed on posters around the gallery. Upon reconvening in plenary session, Larry Pasti of the Forum for Youth Investing and a senior director at Big Picture Approach Consulting moderated a discussion of individual participants' responses to the questions. (Session highlights are presented in Box 3-1.)

NEW YORK CITY DEPARTMENT OF HEALTH AND MENTAL HYGIENE[1]

The New York City DOHMH serves a diverse population of about 8.5 million people, Askew said. For perspective, he noted that the second most populous city in the United States is Los Angeles, with 3.9 million residents, and if New York City were a state, it would be the 12th-largest state in the country.

Division of Family and Child Health

Upon joining the DOHMH in 2014, Askew said, he set out to bring together under one umbrella all of the pieces of the health department that were engaged with children or families. The Division of Family and Child Health was established to improve the health of children, women, and families in New York City, with an emphasis on reducing health disparities and advancing equity. The division's goal is that all of the children, women, and families in New York City recognize their power and are given the opportunity to reach their full health and development potential. The Division of Family and Child Health portfolio includes

- Bureau of Maternal, Infant, and Reproductive Health, overseeing around 120,000 births in New York City every year;
- Bureau of Early Intervention, which spends about $500 million per year on early intervention services and serves about 30,000 to 40,000 children in New York City;
- Office of School Health, which serves about 1.2 million school-age children; and
- Early Childhood Health and Development Unit, which is working to change the culture and the way in which the health department understands, supports, and nurtures babies, infants, and toddlers in New York City.

[1] This section is the rapporteur's synopsis of the presentation by George Askew, and the statements are not endorsed or verified by the National Academies of Sciences, Engineering, and Medicine.

BOX 3-1
Highlights and Main Points Made by Individual Speakers and Participants[a]

- In many states there is a lack of coordinated, state-wide sharing of data across early childhood programs and providers. There are also barriers to Medicaid billing. (Shinn-Brown)
- The program capacity of high-quality early care and education programs is insufficient to meet the demand. (Suarez)
- Child care that is both affordable and accessible must come together with the elements of healthy child care and with equity-rooted change levers to achieve high-quality child care and healthy communities that affect the social determinants of health. (Scott)
- The accelerators that enable collaboration include funding, technical assistance, champions in the community (including the business community), and political will. (Askew, Scott, Shinn-Brown, Suarez)
- The elements of successful collaboration include governance and rules of engagement (clear roles and responsibilities) and a clear, shared understanding of what the collaboration is about. (Pasti)
- There is more to making programs sustainable than the financial aspects; sustainability can also be encouraged by embedding initiatives into existing programs and systems, establishing training competencies, and developing cross-sector collaboration efforts, for example. (Chang, Pasti)
- In mapping needs assessments, geographic information system mapping can be used to examine the current use of existing resources from an equity perspective and to better understand the role of place in the health status and behaviors of the community. The resulting data can be used to drive project investments. The mapping process itself can bring many partners together. (Groginsky, Pasti, Scott, Suarez)

[a] This list is the rapporteur's summary of the main points made by individual speakers and participants (noted in parentheses) and does not reflect any consensus among workshop participants or endorsement by the National Academies of Sciences, Engineering, and Medicine.

Cross-Division Collaboration on Social-Emotional Learning

The Division of Family and Child Health and the Division of Mental Hygiene, both within the DOHMH, are involved in a cross-sector collaboration to integrate mental health consulting on social-emotional learning (SEL) into early care and education classroom sites throughout the city.

Social-emotional development, Askew explained, involves developing the capacity of the child (birth to 5 years of age) to form close and secure adult and peer relationships; to experience, manage, and express a full range of emotions; to explore the environment; and to learn, all in the context of family, community, and culture. SEL is the process through which children and adults acquire the knowledge and skills to recognize and manage emotions, show caring and concern for others, establish positive relationships, make responsible decisions, and handle challenging situations constructively. (He noted that these definitions were adapted from materials developed by Zero to Three.)

The SEL initiative is part of ThriveNYC, which was launched by the First Lady of New York City, Chirlane McCray, as a comprehensive plan to approach mental health and substance misuse in the city.[2] ThriveNYC uses a public health approach to change the way people think about mental health and also the way that the city government and its many partners provide care. The SEL project, Askew said, is based on the "Act early" guiding principle of ThriveNYC, which is to give New Yorkers more tools to weather challenges and to capitalize on opportunities by investing in prevention and early intervention. As a component of ThriveNYC, the SEL project is a cross-system collaboration among the Department of Education (DOE, which oversees the universal pre-K program); the Administration for Children's Services (the city's child welfare system, which handles EarlyLearn, an early childhood/early care and education system that includes the Head Start program); and the DOHMH.

Originally, SEL focused on mental health treatment and referrals, Askew said, but it later changed into a provider of mental health consulting services. This focus on consulting enables the program to build capacity in adults working with children and also to build supports focused on prevention (rather than treatment). This focus changed as a result of the community response—specifically, when it was found that mental health consultation was in higher demand than treatment. The program continues to learn from the needs and responsiveness of the children, and more children will now be served in their early care and education classrooms, where mental health supports are less threatening and more accessible, given the life situations of many of the targeted families. Most of the 30 mental health consultants hold master's degrees in social work or a mental health–related degree (e.g., art therapy). Askew said that this program represents about 50 percent of their workload, with the other 50 percent related to treatment.

The framework for the public health approach to early childhood mental health was adapted from the Georgetown University Framework for Early Childhood Mental Health Consultation, Askew said. The New York City model is intended to build capacity (see Figure 3-1), and the first step is to build supportive environments as well as nurturing and

[2] For a brief overview of ThriveNYC, see https://www1.nyc.gov/assets/operations/downloads/pdf/pmmr2017/thrivenyc.pdf (accessed October 30, 2017).

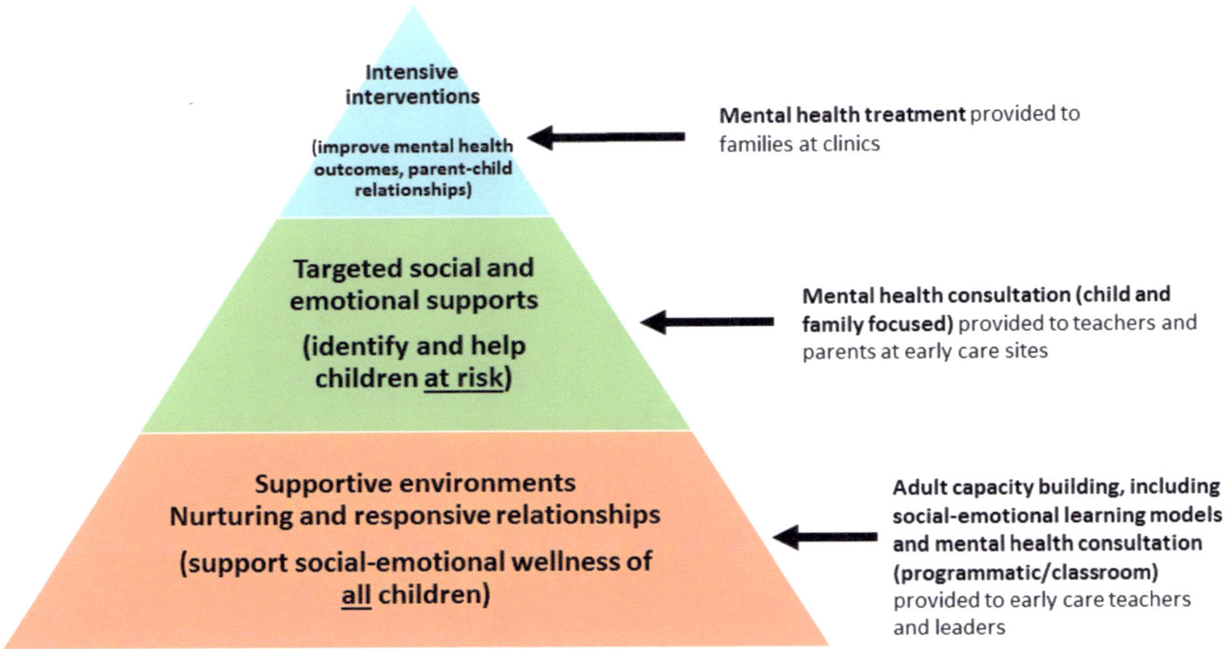

FIGURE 3-1 Public health approach to early childhood mental health.
SOURCES: Askew presentation, September 14, 2017; Bureau of Children, Youth, and Families, New York City Department of Health and Mental Hygiene, 2017.

responsive relationships that will support the social-emotional wellness of all children. This is done through building the capacity of teaching and program staff to foster positive learning and development, to promote each child's social and emotional well-being, and to build relationships with children and communication with parents. The second step is to offer targeted social and emotional supports and to identify those children who need help or are at risk. This is done through specific mental health case consultation. Each mental health consultant carries a case load of about five sites, with a maximum of three classrooms per consultant per site. The number of case-specific consultations will then vary depending upon the needs identified at each site. The New York City model asks that consultants spend one day per week at each early care and education site. The third step is to provide mental health treatment for those children who need it. This is an intensive intervention to alleviate distress and return children to healthy development.

Mental Health Consultation: Accelerators, Challenges, and Community Impact

ThriveNYC has been a program accelerator for the SEL program, Askew said, as all mental health consultants are funded through ThriveNYC. Sustainability has been a challenge, as mental health consultants are not covered through Medicaid. Askew mentioned the possibility of using Medicaid coverage through the First 1,000 Days on Medicaid initiative in New York.[3] Dosage is also an issue. For this approach to be effective, Askew said, the dosage has to be fairly high in order to build the kinds of relationships needed in these environments. Spending only one day per week at each site limits the case load that the mental health consultants can carry. Another challenge is reach. Currently the workforce is reaching about 75 out of 400 sites. The workload of teachers and other adults who are serving children in early learning situations is heavy, and it becomes an obstacle to teachers' full involvement and to their ability to benefit from the intervention of the mental health consultant.

An evaluation is currently being conducted to explore the community impact of the SEL program in the different demographics being served, Askew said. The evaluation is also attempting to look at value in improving teacher well-being as a result of the support and consultations being brought to the environment.

---

[3] See https://www.health.ny.gov/health_care/medicaid/redesign/first_1000.htm (accessed October 30, 2017).

Other Early Care and Education Initiatives at the DOHMH

Askew concluded by briefly describing several other early care and education initiatives at the DOHMH. The Early Intervention program worked with the DOE and the Child Care Bureau to amend the Health Code to ensure that therapists were able to deliver services to children with delays and disabilities in early care and education settings. Askew explained that there had been some issues with care providers not allowing the therapists to enter the early care and education settings. He suggested that states consider what steps might be needed to better facilitate access to children in their natural environments and their least restrictive environments. In response to a question, Askew acknowledged that there is always the question of the ability to enforce the elements of the health code. For any amendments to the health code, he said, there must be some ability to track that it actually gets done.

The DOHMH is also focused on oral health, and it is integrating oral health messaging into its partner newsletters. The results of a Child Dental Survey, which assessed risk and prevention behaviors for tooth decay among children, led the DOHMH to launch an early childhood dental caries campaign. The department has also developed, Askew said, a policy proposal to amend the child care regulations and the health code to mandate tooth brushing at all child care centers in New York City.

The DOHMH's Division of Prevention and Primary Care has a variety of programs focused on nutrition, healthy eating, physical activity, and active design, Askew said. For example, the Eat Well, Play Hard program is a nutrition education program led by registered dieticians in group child care centers. The program reaches approximately 100 centers in the city and targets children ages 3 and 4 years old as well as caregivers and child care staff. The Farm to Preschool program provides opportunities for parents and staff to purchase a box of local produce at child care centers, offers nutrition education and cooking demonstrations for adults, and provides teachers with a curriculum to engage children in gardening.

Finally, the Active Design in Early Child Care Settings program provides active design mini-grants to early child care centers located in low-income neighborhoods throughout the five boroughs. The goal of these mini-grants, Askew said, is for sites to purchase low-cost enhancements that increase active play in the outdoor spaces at their centers (e.g., gardens, circulation routes, loose toys). These are just some of the ways the New York City DOHMH is working to integrate health into the early care and education setting, he concluded.

HEAD START AS A LEVER TO IMPROVE POPULATION HEALTH

Head Start is a federally funded program serving pregnant women and children, from birth to kindergarten entry, who are at or below the federal poverty guideline, Shinn-Brown said. Federal requirements for the program are intended to support the whole child, and Head Start is meant to be a comprehensive child and family development program.

Health is a critical factor in early childhood education and school readiness. Children who come to school with, for example, teeth that hurt, runny noses and earaches, or trauma in their lives and behavioral dysfunction in their families do not learn as well as children who come to school without those challenges, Shinn-Brown said. Head Start is focused on primary prevention and health promotion, and the program gathers data to inform its practice and ensure that it is supporting children's health. Head Start is federally mandated to provide screening, referral, follow-up, integrated health education, and ongoing observation and assessment, she said. Head Start programs are able, through specific processes, to use Medicaid funds and private insurance funds to offset the costs of providing these services; Head Start itself is the payer of last resort.

Supporting Health Equity

Head Start supports health equity. It is more cost effective for families to have good health care than it is for them to suffer the ill effects of poor health care, Shinn-Brown said. She raised concerns about cost containment measures within state systems that tend to force families out of care, instead of bringing them into care.

One approach to fostering equity is addressing family health literacy. Shinn-Brown referred participants to the work of Ariella Herman of the University of California, Los Angeles, Health Care Institute.[4] The Health Care Institute's approach to health literacy education is used by Head Start programs. Shinn-Brown said that Herman's groundbreaking work has demonstrated the importance of health literacy in helping parents be good consumers of health care, in reducing lost time for illness and absenteeism both for parents and their children, and in reducing emergency department visits and increasing connections with medical and dental homes.

Shinn-Brown said that Head Start also supports health equity through family advocates who work individually with families to help them set

---

[4] For information, see http://www.anderson.ucla.edu/centers/price-center-for-entrepreneurship-and-innovation/for-professionals/health-care-institute (accessed October 30, 2017).

goals that support positive health outcomes. The family advocates emphasize health promotion and disease prevention, and they work with families to help them maintain their insurance coverage, overcome barriers to access (especially in rural areas), and keep appointments.

Developing Relationships with the Community and the Health System

Every Head Start program must conduct a community assessment of the factors that affect the health of the population it serves, Shinn-Brown said. Each Head Start program also convenes a health services advisory committee, which is a multidisciplinary group of professionals, including parents, who help the program make decisions about services, referrals, resources, and policies and procedures.

Head Start partners with many different types of providers to supplement Head Start funding with community resources. These providers include federally qualified health centers; hospital systems; mental health providers; community health departments; the Supplemental Nutrition Program for Women, Infants, and Children (WIC); and others. Shinn-Brown said that Head Start struggles to provide mental health services in her state, and she emphasized the importance of mental health services for young children who experience trauma and of trauma-informed practices to support young children and their families.

Providing the Required Health Screenings

Head Start programs are required to provide a range of health screenings, using valid and reliable tools. Vision is tested using an instrument-based screening approach and symbol sets. As an example of how valuable these screening practices can be, Shinn-Brown said that OACAC Head Start serves just under 1,000 children in its 10-county service area in Missouri, and last year 156 children were referred for a vision concern. Head Start does not offer diagnoses, but instead it screens and refers families to their primary care provider for follow-up. Of the 156 children referred, 136 received glasses. This means, she said, that more than 10 percent of the children in OACAC Head Start—children who had a medical home—had not been identified as having a significant vision concern early in their childhood experience. Other screenings include hearing, dental, developmental, sensory, behavioral and mental health, nutrition status, and injury prevention. OACAC Head Start partners with Parents as Teachers, a home visit–based curriculum model for child development, to provide developmental screens. Shinn-Brown noted that sensory screening can be a challenge when a child has a sensory processing disorder, for example, or autism spectrum issues. As mentioned, Head Start programs may use Medicaid and private insurance as a reimbursement stream and may use Medicaid reimbursement to offset the cost of these types of screenings. OACAC Head Start contracts with a local physician, who writes standing orders for all of the required screenings so that they are billable. Shinn-Brown said that Medicaid reimbursement also allows her Head Start program to fund three full-time counselors on staff as well as a full-time nurse and a part-time nurse. She said that the state is continuing to work through the transition from a Medicaid fee-for-service model to a managed care system and is lagging behind in terms of best practices.

Challenges

Shinn-Brown highlighted several challenges Head Start faces. Many states, including Missouri, lack coordinated, state-wide early childhood systems, she said. For example, there are barriers to Head Start and WIC providers sharing information about children who are nutritionally at risk (above the 95th percentile or below the 5th percentile). There are now ongoing efforts to find ways to share information instead of duplicating efforts, she said.

Another challenge is that, especially in rural areas, there is an over-reliance on the parent report in the health system to meet the Medicaid Early and Periodic Screening, Diagnostic, and Treatment requirements, Shinn-Brown said. She observed that there is often a "wait and see" attitude among pediatricians in the more rural areas when it comes to developmental issues. This results in children not being referred for services when they could have been eligible for Missouri's First Steps early intervention services for children ages birth to 3 years (under Part C of the Individuals with Disabilities Education and Improvement Act), she added.

Access to appropriate behavioral health supports for very young children, including to mental health professionals trained in a trauma-informed care approach, is also lacking, Shinn-Brown said. Health equity and access affect suspensions and expulsions in young children, particularly young children of color. Until there is a more effective way of supporting young children with a trauma-informed care approach, she said, young children will continue to be expelled from classrooms and then bounce from program to program until they land at Head Start's door. This is a complicated and difficult situation, she said, and she emphasized the need to support all child care providers so that they in turn are able to support all children.

HEALTH, ACCESS, AND AFFORDABILITY IN CHILD CARE

Child Care Aware of America is a national nonprofit membership organization for local child care resource and referral agencies.[5] In many states, Scott said, these agencies are responsible for consumer education and for connecting parents and families with child care in their area, which involves getting to know families and what they need. Resource and referral agencies also conduct much of the training and professional development done within states to help improve the child care workforce, and they are also involved in policy development and advocacy.

As senior director for health policy at Child Care Aware, Scott said, she is focused on how to make child care settings as healthy as possible. She listed some of the current state-level early care and education priorities that the member agencies are working on. In Minnesota, for example, one of the priority issues is addressing a shortage of licensed care providers. In Maryland, the current priority is increasing the Child Care Subsidy Program budget to help the lowest-income families access child care.

Another priority area for the agencies is the implementation of the reauthorized Child Care Development Block Grant, in light of the many new requirements for such grants. Scott highlighted three key aspects of the reauthorized block grant: it authorizes the Child Care and Development Fund, which provides federal funds for states to disburse child care subsidies for low-income families; it establishes baseline standards for child care systems that states must meet in order to receive this funding; and the receipt of funding obligates states to invest in improving the quality of child care. Scott noted that only one in every ten children who are eligible for federal child care subsidies actually receive them.

Establishing Standards

Prior to the reauthorization of the block grant, Scott said, states varied widely with regard to basic health and safety standards, and she referred participants to two Child Care Aware reports, *We Can Do Better* and *Leaving Children to Chance*, which chronicle state policies on health and safety requirements for child care.[6] At the time of the reports (2013 and 2012, respectively), most states had requirements for basic health and safety, but only 16 states met all of the 10 health and 10 safety practices recommended by pediatric experts. Scott also mentioned the Child Care Licensing Database, which compares state licensing regulations to the recommended

---

[5] See http://childcareaware.org (accessed October 30, 2017).

[6] These reports and other advocacy and policy resources are available at http://usa.childcareaware.org/advocacy-public-policy/child-care-and-development-block-grant-ccdbg (accessed October 30, 2017).

standards outlined by the Administration for Children and Families in the report *Caring for Our Children Basics*.[7]

Investing in Quality

As noted, the reauthorized block grant requires states to invest in activities that improve the quality of child care. The amount of funds that must be spent on quality improvement increases over the course of implementation of the reauthorized block grant, Scott said, and by 2021 states will be required to set aside a total of 12 percent of their block grant funds for quality-improvement activities (9 percent, plus an additional 3 percent specifically for infant/toddler quality-improvement activities). Under the program requirements there are many different quality-improvement activities that states can spend block grant funding on. Scott mentioned several examples, including basic health and safety training for all child care providers (including health, nutrition, physical activity, and obesity prevention); consumer education, including websites with information on quality, best practices, and support services (e.g., WIC, Medicaid); and the incorporation of healthy active living into quality rating and improvement systems.

Healthy Child Care, Healthy Communities

Scott described the Healthy Child Care, Health Communities Project as an example of how Child Care Aware partners with state systems to help them include health in their state child care plans. Child Care Aware has developed recommended language for states to use in drafting their state plans. She noted that Alabama used this language to make public comment recommendations on its initial state plan. In addition, a toolkit was created to help states develop messaging that resonates with child care providers and the public to increase acceptance of change. Focus groups on staff health and wellness were held in order to understand the ways in which the new policies being enacted were affecting the behaviors of the child care providers themselves. Scott noted, for example, that providers are modeling healthy behavior in front of the children (e.g., not drinking soda), which is good for them as well as for the children.

Geographic information system mapping is done to examine the current use of existing resources from an equity perspective. These data

[7] The Child Care Aware of America Child Care State Licensing Database is available at http://licensingdatabase.usa.child careaware.org. The Administration for Children and Families report *Caring for Our Children Basics* is available at https://www.acf.hhs.gov/sites/default/files/ecd/caring_for_our_children_basics.pdf (accessed October 30, 2017).

are then used to drive project investments and engage stakeholders to develop cross-sector solutions. The Alabama Farm to Early Care and Education program, for example, is exploring the relationship between family child care providers and proximity to farmers, with regard to opportunities for the procurement of fresh local foods. In New York, breastfeeding-friendly communities are being mapped. In Indiana, mapping is being done of where there is access to safe spaces to play in community revitalization neighborhood grantees, to identify where investments are needed, and to encourage care providers to use those spaces for active play.

In closing, Scott described her theory of change (see Figure 3-2). It is not enough to have healthy spaces, she said. Affordable and accessible child care, elements of healthy child care, and equity-rooted change levers must come together to achieve high-quality child care and healthy communities, which in turn affect the social determinants of health.

PROSPER LINCOLN

Prosper Lincoln is a community initiative that seeks to transform Lincoln, Nebraska, into a thriving community for people to live, work, and play, where there is equitable opportunity for all residents to have the income, education, and resources they need to be successful, Suarez said.[8] Lincoln, the capital of Nebraska, is home to about 280,000 people. The unemployment rate is 2.6 percent, the crime rate is low, and there is affordable housing. In 2014 the first Lincoln Vital Signs report was released, examining the statistics and demographics in Lincoln. The report concluded that Lincoln does many things exceptionally well and should be proud of its accomplishments and the quality of life, Suarez said. However, it was also found that a growing proportion of Lincoln's population faces real need and that Lincoln's children are particularly vulnerable. Prosper Lincoln was begun as the community's response to these findings, with the overall goal of addressing youth success, economic prosperity, and quality of life. Eight key sectors have been involved in the development of the community agenda: (1) nonprofit organizations, networks, and cultural centers; (2) businesses; (3) neighborhoods and the general public; (4) the public sector; (5) the faith community; (6) anchor institutions (e.g., universities, hospitals); (7) K–12 education; and (8) philanthropy and donors. Together, these sectors are working to improve the health and prosperity of Lincoln.

Also in 2014, the Community Health Endowment of Lincoln undertook a mapping project to better understand the role of place in the

[8] For more information, see https://www.prosperlincoln.org (accessed October 30, 2017).

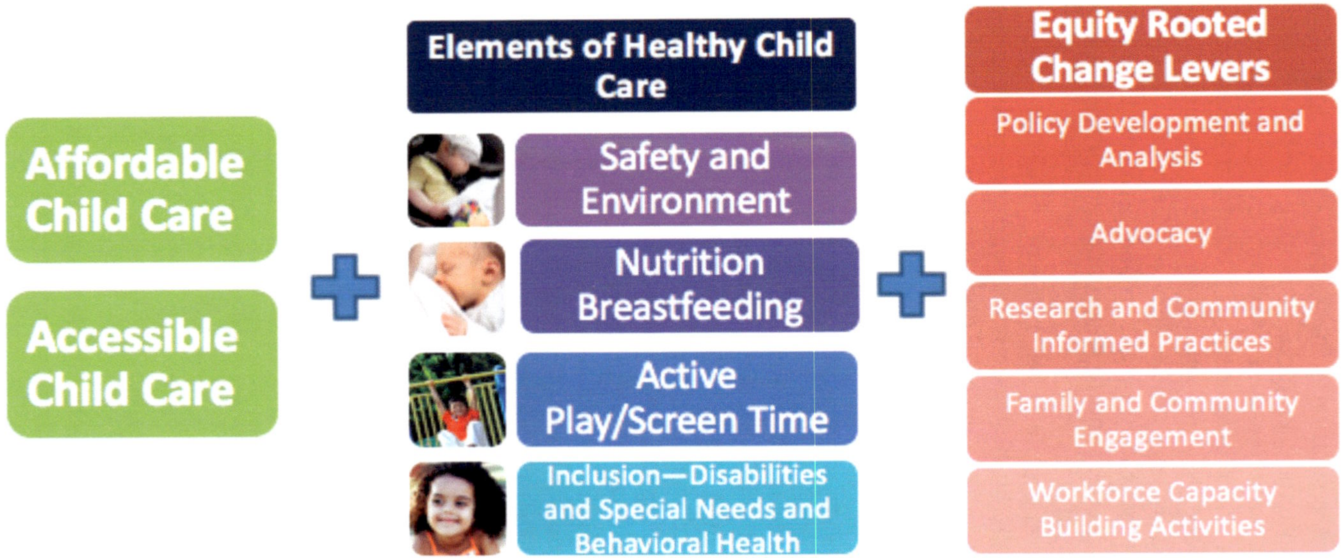
Affordable Child Care
Accessible Child Care
Elements of Healthy Child Care
Safety and Environment
Nutrition Breastfeeding
Active Play/Screen Time
Inclusion—Disabilities and Special Needs and Behavioral Health
Equity Rooted Change Levers
Policy Development and Analysis
Advocacy
Research and Community Informed Practices
Family and Community Engagement
Workforce Capacity Building Activities

FIGURE 3-2 Theory of change to achieve high-quality child care and healthy communities.
SOURCE: Scott presentation, September 14, 2017.

health status and behaviors in the community. The results showed that place matters. Depending on where one lives in Lincoln, Suarez said, life expectancy varies by as much as 20 years or more.

To begin to address these issues of quality of life in Lincoln, funding priorities were identified, and early childhood was targeted for health, wellness, and prevention interventions. High-quality early childhood development and learning affect children in both the short term and long term, Suarez said. The foundation for later learning, behavior, and health is dependent upon the quality of early learning and care. Interventions and support are most effective in the first 3 years of life, but many of the children who need help and support the most are not receiving it. In Lincoln, approximately 65 percent of the most vulnerable children ages 3 to 5 are not enrolled in preschool programs. The percent of children in poverty in Lincoln increased by 78 percent between 2008 and 2015, and more than 12,100 children (1 in 5) are now living in poverty. The program capacity of high-quality early care and education programs is insufficient to meet this demand.

Prosper Lincoln Strategic Plan for Early Childhood

The Prosper Lincoln community agenda was developed around three priorities: early childhood, employment skills, and innovation. Strategic plans were developed over the course of 12 months, through an intensive community engagement process, and the implementation of the plans began in August 2016. The overall desired outcome of the strategic plan for early childhood, Suarez explained, is to reach the Prosper Lincoln goal of nurturing every child on the path to success. The specific goal is for all children to be kindergarten ready. Work is ongoing with the public school system to identify measures of literacy and numeracy and to determine how to measure SEL learning and executive function.

Suarez said that the "kindergarten ready" goal also implies that schools and communities are ready to meet the needs of the children. In this regard, a Community Early Childhood System of Care self-assessment was conducted. Providers and parents were asked about their perspectives on schools, family resources, health, and early childhood mental health. Provider and parent responses were compared to identify gaps and develop priorities for action, which led to the convening of three workgroups focused on the following topics:

- **Quality care and education.** Data and mapping studies inform the work of this group. More resources are needed, Suarez said, so that children from low-income families have access to high-quality early care and education.

- **Comprehensive health, including early childhood mental health.** This group is convening public sessions to develop a vision of what Lincoln wants for its children. Specifically, it is asking: What are the essential community elements needed to ensure that children and their families are safe, heathy, and kindergarten ready? What systems of data collection are needed to better track children's progress from birth to kindergarten and to make sure that stakeholders who support children are all on the same page?
- **Communication and messaging.** Communication and messaging is a very important part of the strategy, Suarez said. She noted that the mayor of Lincoln met with about 100 business leaders who are coming to the table because they see the potential return on investment in a healthier community.

Programs

Suarez shared an example of a parent education program at a school with a very large immigrant and refugee population. The program was designed so that parents could explore a topic related to children with a focus on early childhood, learn about books they can share with their children, and practice a learning activity they can do at home with their children. Suarez said that because English is not the first language for many of these families, the presentation includes many visual examples. For example, the idea that protective factors help create strong families was likened to the use of insulation in a house. Concepts such as executive function can be difficult to communicate, but graphics can help to get the message across, she said. There are also interpreters available to help translate the presentation. Programs include a book and a play activity and emphasize the importance of pretend play as part of learning. Parents try the activity during the program, and they discuss examples of what they can talk about with their children at home. The activity adds enjoyment and levity to the program as well as providing parents with a play activity they can do at home. There is also interactive discussion of various topics, such as keeping families strong, parental resilience, and concrete support systems, with parents sharing their ideas.

Prosper Lincoln continues to measure the outcomes of its work, Suarez said, and has metrics in place for its early childhood strategies.

DISCUSSION

Moderator Chang observed that discussions of sustainability are often focused on financial sustainability. She suggested that one should consider sustainability in more than just the financial aspects. As discussed in the examples in both sessions thus far, embedding programs into state systems, establishing training competencies, and collaborating across sectors are non-financial approaches to help sustain programs. Following up on the many examples of collaborations discussed, Chang asked panelists to consider accelerators (i.e., catalysts) that might enable collaboration as well as any barriers to partnerships that might need to be addressed.

Accelerators and Barriers to Partnerships

Askew reiterated that a key accelerator for the SEL initiative has been that it is part of ThriveNYC, which is championed by the First Lady of New York City. Having the backing of the city government can be a great advantage, he said, and political will is a strong driver of activity. Scott agreed with the power of political will. She said that from her experience across 68 partnerships, those partnerships that do not have political will behind them must rely on money and technical assistance to pave their way. Funding brings people to the table and allows them to have conversations they would not typically be able to have. Shinn-Brown agreed with the need for champions in the community. OACAC Head Start looks for children's champions who will help move an initiative forward. She said that the Mayor's Commission for Children in Springfield, Missouri, which includes members of the business community, is one such group of champions, and Head Start has leveraged the commission's talents and connections. The business community is a key accelerator, Suarez agreed, and she said it is important to make sure that community becomes part of the fabric of the work.

One of the basic barriers to collaboration, Askew said, is that it is hard. Breaking down silos and getting people to "leave their egos at the door" and accept a genuine partnership can be difficult, even among colleagues who like each other and who generally work well together. Scott suggested that unintended consequences of policies can be barriers to partnerships. Shinn-Brown observed that there are challenges when an administration is committed but the shared vision has not been firmly and adequately articulated downstream to the staff who are doing the daily work to resolve issues of competing priorities. Suarez suggested that one barrier is that people simply may not fully comprehend the importance of a child's early years as the foundational time for health and healthy behaviors. A significant, ongoing educational component is needed to ensure that people understand that this is where attention is needed.

Pasti observed that much of the discussion has been centered on external collaboration, and he asked about cross-sector collaboration within a large organization, such as the New York City DOHMH. Askew said that there are often long-standing silos that can be difficult to break down, but efforts are being made. He cited his efforts to bring together all of the people working on early childhood health and development across multiple areas within the health department to share information and avoid duplication.

Additional Gaps and Opportunities

Carrie Bateman of the New York City DOE pointed to disability as one gap in the intersection between health and education. New York City currently has 270,000 students with disabilities, which is about 21 percent of the total student population, she said, noting that the national rate is about 13 percent.

Dave Kindig of the University of Wisconsin–Madison asked about the degree to which nonprofit hospitals (which are required to do community benefit as a condition of their tax-exempt status) are addressing the early care and education resource gaps. Scott replied that she had heard anecdotally that it is part of the conversation. Chang said that a number of children's hospitals are focused on this, mentioning in particular Nemours Children's Health System, Atlanta Children's Hospital, and Cincinnati Children's Hospital.

Kindig suggested that one role for those in population health will be finding ways in which the health care system and public health can help the early care and education sector achieve its goals. There is a co-benefit to both sectors. Askew added that it is incumbent upon those in health to partner with those in housing, parks, education, and other sectors in order to address the issues known to be social determinants of health.

GALLERY WALK REFLECTIONS

Following the panel discussion, participants moved to the gallery to consider the following:

- How can cross-sector collaboration in early care and education and health be accelerated? What do organizations need to collaborate more effectively?
- What are the main barriers to collaboration, and what are solutions to overcome them?
- What can be learned from other cross-sector collaborations that could inform early care and education and health interactions?
- What new insights can participants offer?

Upon reconvening, Pasti summarized the responses to the questions posed in the gallery and moderated the discussion. He observed that much of the workshop conversation around collaboration was focused on children from birth to age 3. He emphasized the need to engage those working beyond the birth to age 3 segment in conversations about common terms, programs, and practices in order to better enable support of young people as they grow throughout their life spans. To increase the chances that the efforts are sustainable, collaboration across the age span will be important. Reflecting on the comments that were made in the gallery, Pasti drew out three main themes: trust, infrastructure, and leveraging the existing work.

- **Trust.** Pasti noted that the issue of trust was raised during the discussions of community engagement. Trust is also essential for collaboration. Some of the comments noted the issue of "turf" as a barrier to collaboration. It was also noted that, when engaging in new collaborations, it is important to pay attention to the history of collaboration in the particular community. Building relationships was highlighted as an important element of collaboration. The element of trust is also critical to family engagement, Pasti observed. Family engagement is not just talking to a family's members about what their needs are, but it is also having them actively involved in the solutions, interventions, and evaluations, thereby fostering community ownership of the issues and outcomes. One aspect of collaboration that is often overlooked is youth engagement, as the focus is often on the parents. Pasti mentioned an example from one of the communities involved in the 100 Million Healthier Lives initiative. A group of high school students who had learned about a continuous improvement model felt that model was important and wanted to share it, so they started teaching sixth-graders the continuous improvement model. This raises the question of how to tap into youth and engage young people in more meaningful ways, Pasti said. He mentioned the concept of two-generation approaches that address the needs of both parents and children (i.e., the whole family).
- **Infrastructure.** Several comments posted focused on the infrastructure or the "ingredients" needed to make collaboration work. Governance and the rules of engagement are important, Pasti said. This includes treating one another with respect and making sure that the roles and responsibilities are clear. It is also important to "get down to basics" and establish exactly what it is that the collaboration is for (e.g., money, sharing information, training and professional development, data, evaluation, technical assistance, resources).
- **Leveraging the existing work.** Comments were made about the need to pay attention to the existing work. As mentioned earlier,

> sustainability is not only about money; it can also stem from embedding initiatives into existing programs and systems. An example was posted about leveraging health sector regulations around community health needs assessment and community health improvement plans. How can early care and education and health initiatives be built into those plans to provide sustainability? Can early education and health initiatives be tied into other "cradle to career" programs? There were also comments about the use of common terms. Pasti noted that the same words cannot always be used across programs, as particular terminology might be required by regulation or statute. Conversations are needed to ensure translation and understanding of what is included when a particular term is used.

One participant emphasized that leadership is essential to collaboration. She suggested that there is a knowledge gap among those in leadership positions who make decisions about funding and financing within the state Medicaid offices, within managed care and health insurance companies, and within health agencies concerning issues involving young children. Those in leadership positions do not think about young children, she suggested, perhaps because they are not the primary drivers of cost in their decisions. She mentioned New York's First 1,000 Days on Medicaid Initiative as a step toward spreading the message about the need to focus on early child development. Pasti agreed and mentioned the need to invite a broad array of stakeholders to the table and to not make assumptions about what they do or do not know. In addition, training is generally attended by those with the same background or responsibilities. There are opportunities to invite others beyond the early child care and health sectors, such as those working in child welfare. Pasti suggested that cross-system professional development can help break down the barriers between disciplines and foster understanding of what is important to each organization. Start small, he suggested, and invite other stakeholders to existing trainings.

Elizabeth Groginsky, the assistant superintendent for early learning in the District of Columbia, referred participants to the program Our Children, Our Community, Our Change and to the Early Development Instrument, a population-based measure of school readiness.[9] The program has mapped the city at the neighborhood-cluster level for health, development, and school readiness at the pre-K/age 4 level. Additional data, such as violent crime and assets, were overlaid on the readiness maps. The mapping process brought many partners together, she said,

[9] See http://www.raisedc.org/ourchildren (accessed October 30, 2017).

and the mayor encouraged all of the state district agencies to take a look at it. Such population-based data can help sectors come together and share data that could add to the conversation, she said. There is also a facilitator's guide that leads people through how to bring cross-sector local community partners together to facilitate conversation and begin to take action on the data. The goal is to change those conditions in communities that are affecting young children entering school so they are ready to learn. Pasti added that these mapping data also help to facilitate conversations about equity. There are some areas, for example, that have high assets but low scores. The data allow for consideration of the deeper issues that affect students.

4

Potential Policy Challenges and Opportunities

The early childhood workforce includes people employed in a variety of roles and in different types of settings, all working on behalf of young children, said Jacqueline Jones, the president and chief executive officer of the Foundation for Child Development and session moderator. There is now an extraordinary effort by those in the early childhood field as well as those in the philanthropic community and government to better understand the needs of the early childhood workforce and to support them through professional learning opportunities and improved compensation, Jones said. The early childhood workforce is generally poorly compensated, which presents challenges for maintaining staffing. Every state has a set of competencies for early childhood teachers, Jones said, but the requirements vary from state to state. There are two national certifications in the field of early childhood education, the Child Development Associate credential for entry-level teachers and the National Board for Professional Teaching Standards for accomplished teachers. However, Jones added, in the middle tier, which accounts for most of the early childhood workforce, there is no national certification that defines what should be known and what skills should be required.

In this session the panel considered policy challenges and opportunities at the intersection of early care and education and health as they relate to such issues as finance, workforce, and equity. Marcy Whitebook, the director of the Center for Study of Child Care Employment at the University of California, Berkeley, who spoke remotely via phone, described the early care and education system in the United States, including workforce and economic issues. Rolf Grafwallner, the program director for early childhood initiatives at the Council of Chief State School Officers, discussed incorporating social-emotional learning (SEL) into state policies and into school and early childhood curricula. Gloria Higgins, the executive director of Executives Partnering to Invest in Children (EPIC), discussed opportunities to engage the business community in supporting early care and education. Aly Richards, the chief executive officer of the Permanent Fund for Vermont's Children, described the various approaches being used to reach the organization's goal of high-quality, affordable early care and learning for all who need it in Vermont by 2025. Finally, Danielle Ewen of EducationCounsel, LLC, discussed intentional and opportunistic approaches to changing policy and practice at the intersection of early care and education and health.

Following the presentations and discussion, participants moved to the adjacent gallery to reflect on the panel discussion with other attendees and to consider specific questions that were posed on posters around the gallery. After the participants reconvened in plenary session, a discussion of the responses to the questions was moderated by Paula Lantz, the associate dean for academic affairs and a professor of public policy at the Gerald R. Ford School of Public Policy of the University of Michigan. (Session highlights are presented in Box 4-1.)

POLICY HIGHLIGHTS AT THE INTERSECTION OF HEALTH AND EARLY CARE AND EDUCATION[1]

The current early care and education system in the United States is less than optimal, Whitebook said. The scientific evidence about human development, early experiences, and long-term health outcomes that has been amassed over recent decades underscores the individual and societal long-term consequences of tolerating what is a suboptimal and, in many ways, dangerous status quo for some children, she continued. From its inception, the Head Start program has considered the health needs of children and has seen that those needs went hand in hand with the educational focus of the program. That is not the case for most early care and education services, however. The health and well-being of early education teachers is also fundamental to the quality of their teaching, but many experience burnout and other occupational health and safety issues.

There are clear areas of progress, Whitebook said, but there are systematic barriers to efforts to coordinate between health and early child-

[1] This section is the rapporteur's synopsis of the presentation by Marcy Whitebook, and the statements are not endorsed or verified by the National Academies of Sciences, Engineering, and Medicine.

BOX 4-1
Highlights and Main Points Made by Individual Speakers and Participants[a]

- The structure of the early care and education system reinforces inequities because children do not necessarily have equal access to high-quality services. (Whitebook)
- Significant brain architecture is built early in life, and the return on investment from early childhood development interventions is well established. However, the pattern of investments in children—as well as the compensation structure for early care and education providers—is inversely related to the brain development curve of young children. (Richards, Whitebook)
- Economic insecurity is a significant concern among early care and education providers and can cause considerable stress, affecting teacher effectiveness and their physical and mental health. (Whitebook)
- Employers are motivated to support early childhood education, in part because they recognize the impact that it has on the future availability of skilled employees. They are also motivated by the business costs associated with employee child care issues and also the benefits, in the form of tax-advantaged opportunities, to companies that engage in early care and education issues. (Higgins)
- Most children are in some form of out-of-home care, and an accessible, high-quality, affordable system of care could provide a safe environment, a huge population for primary prevention activities, and a cost-effective, streamlined platform in which to co-administer other health services. (Richards)

[a] This list is the rapporteur's summary of the main points made by individual speakers and participants (noted in parentheses) and does not reflect any consensus among workshop participants or endorsement by the National Academies of Sciences, Engineering, and Medicine.

hood care. As a case example, she described First 5 California, an initiative to improve early childhood outcomes in the areas of health and nutrition, early literacy and language development, high-quality child care, and smoking cessation. The program was launched in 1998 and is funded by a voter-approved tobacco tax. First 5 California brought together health and early childhood practitioners from every county to determine how best to use the resources from the tobacco tax. An immediate challenge, Whitebrook said, was that the different disciplines had long been siloed, and there was a lot of "talking past each other." This stemmed, she said, from the complexity of each discipline, socialization and terminology that differed from profession to profession, and differences between the institutions where services were delivered. Communication was further complicated by different assumptions and different levels of status and authority. Although progress has been made, Whitebrook said, these issues still need to be taken into account when those from different disciplines work together today. The First 5 California collaboration was strengthened by shared issues, she said. Both the health and the early childhood communities had tended to divorce child policy issues from their wider environment of relationships. Together they began to craft more multi-generational approaches. There was a focus on co-location of services, bringing mental health and other health practitioners into child care centers and homes, and thinking more holistically about the families and the communities in which children develop. In the process, Whitebook said, each discipline gained more respect for and understanding of the unique contributions made by other disciplines.

U.S. Early Care and Education System

The benefits of high-quality early care and education are often discussed in terms of "how it can ameliorate the effects of poverty, level the playing field for young children, provide support to families, and promote healthy behaviors and development," Whitebook said. Those promises are coming to fruition in most other industrialized countries, Whitebook added, but despite tremendous effort, most children in the United States are not experiencing those benefits. Too often, she said, the design and financing of the U.S. early care and education system causes poverty for many families because of the cost. The system may ameliorate the cost burden for some families, but not for all who need help. The way that the early care and education system is structured reinforces and sometimes accentuates inequities, Whitebook added, because children do not necessarily have equal access to high-quality services. Economic stress undermines the health and well-being of the adults in children's lives, including their parents, as well as of the poorly paid teachers and care providers.

An underlying cause of the state of early care and education is that the United States does not have a system of early care and education in which the government, either national or state, has assumed leadership responsibility for ensuring that services are available, affordable, and of high quality for all children and families. Early care and education is not defined as a public good in the same way that K–12 education is, Whitebook said. Rather, it is usually considered a private family responsibility. The structure assumes that the demand for early care will be met by a diverse and centralized private market. This structure contributes to inequity, Whitebook explained, because those with a greater ability to pay typically obtain the best services in a private market. In essence, early care and education has been monetized and is treated as a commodity. Except for in a handful of communities, she said, early care and education is not treated as part of the infrastructure of the educational system.

The federal government does intervene in the market on behalf of low-income families by offering each state a limited public subsidy based on the size of its low-income child population, Whitebook said. There are not enough resources, however, and only a fraction of children who qualify for subsidized child care are currently receiving it. For example, in 2014, 6.4 million children under the age of 6 lived in low-income working families, but only 1.41 million received a child care subsidy. Similarly, there is limited provision of state-funded public preschool, and less than half of the children who qualify for Head Start nationally are being served. Whitebook said that the United States devotes a much smaller percentage of its gross domestic product than other industrialized countries to early childhood services (see Figure 4-1). The United States also puts a smaller amount of its gross domestic product into health services than other industrialized countries. As a result, early childhood services are under-resourced compared with those in many other countries.

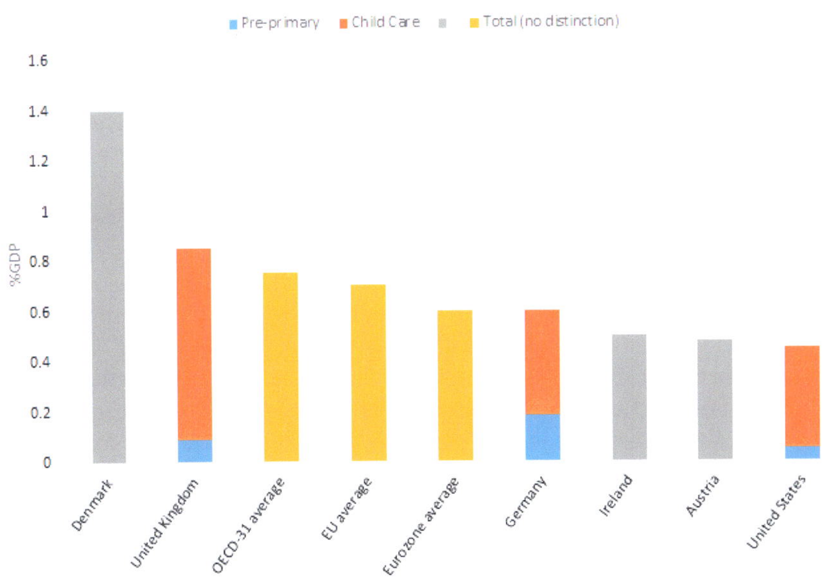

FIGURE 4-1 Public spending on early care and education (2013 data).
NOTE: EU = European Union; GDP = gross domestic product; OECD = Organisation for Economic Co-operation and Development.
SOURCES: Whitebook presentation, September 14, 2017, adapted from the OECD Family Database. See http://www.oecd.org/els/soc/PF3_1_Public_spending_on_childcare_and_early_education.pdf (accessed October 30, 2017).

Impact of Early Care and Education on Health and Well-Being

Whitebook noted that much of the conversation in the early care and education field has focused on the types of qualifications that should be required of people working with young children (e.g., foundational knowledge of early development, bachelor's degree with specialized training). The 2015 Institute of Medicine (IOM) and National Research Council (NRC) consensus report on transforming the early childhood workforce also highlighted the importance of the well-being of the adults in children's lives, she said. The day-to-day interactions between caregivers and young children builds the initial architecture of the children's brains and establishes their patterns of thinking and feeling. As such, the health and well-being of the people providing those early experiences are critical, Whitebook said. The IOM and NRC consensus report states the following:

> Adults who are under-informed, underprepared, or subject to chronic stress themselves may contribute to children's experiences of adversity and stress and undermine their development and learning. (IOM and NRC, 2015, p. 4)

The Economics of Early Care and Education

Early care and education policies in the United States can create stress for parents from the start, Whitebook said. In addition to the stress of arranging and paying for child care, most parents do not have paid family leave. They are left to choose between leaving their babies in care at a very young age or losing job security and income during this crucial period for the family. The burden is greatest on low-income families, she said. The cost burden for families is significant. Fifty-four percent of families pay more than 10 percent of their income for child care. In 32 states and the District of Columbia, center-based infant care costs are greater than one-third of a typical preschool worker's earnings. For child care teachers who are also parents of young children, the stresses brought on by their low wages and high care costs are even greater.

The lack of sufficient financing of subsidies for early care and education means that rates for care are usually held low, so that more children can be served, Whitebook said. Because so many parents have difficulty covering the cost of care, there is significant market pressure to keep the cost low as well. It is the early care teachers who end up assuming the burden of this lack of financing through their low wages. The 2015 IOM and NRC workforce consensus report emphasized that most early educators suffer from deeply substandard compensation, which fails to reward their investments in education and

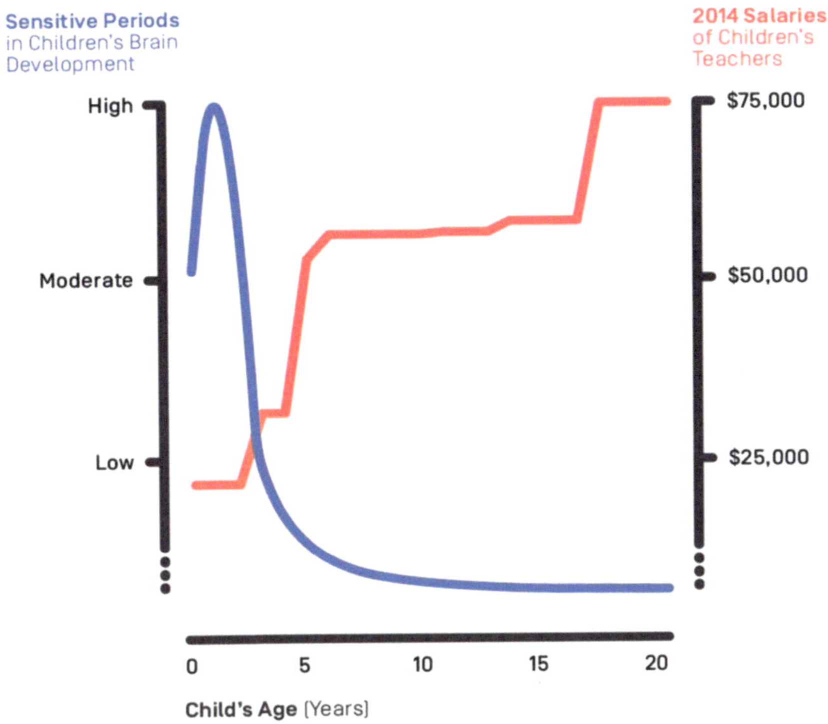

FIGURE 4-2 Inverse relationship between the sensitive learning periods in child brain development and educator compensation.
SOURCES: Whitebook presentation, September 14, 2017; Thompson and Nelson, 2001; Whitebook et al., 2014.

training and which ultimately threatens their well-being. Whitebook told participants that a related National Academies study on financing high-quality early care and education in the United States is currently under way.[2]

Educational interventions during the early years have the highest returns on investment because they provide the highest returns on learning, Whitebook said. The compensation structure of the early care and education system is inverse to the brain development curve (see Figure 4-2). People often assume that wages are low because those workers have not invested in education and training. Actually, about one-third of

[2] Information about this National Academies consensus study and resulting report (released in 2018) can be found at http://sites.nationalacademies.org/DBASSE/BCYF/Finance_ECE/index.htm (accessed accessed August 9, 2018).

the early childhood workforce (including those working with infants and toddlers in center-based care) have college degrees. Of those working with 3- to 5-year-old children, close to 40 percent have college degrees.

Whitebook said that much of the conversation in the early care and education field has focused on the types of qualifications that should be required of all people working with young children (e.g., foundational knowledge of early development, bachelor's degree with specialized training), while little attention has been focused on the need for professional support and appropriate financial rewards.

Wages for some early care and education teachers are very low compared to wages for teachers working with kindergarten age and early elementary age children, Whitebook said. In 2012 the average annual salary for an early care and education teacher with a bachelor's degree or higher was about $27,000 for those working with children ages birth to 3 years and about $29,000 for those working with ages 3 to 5 years. Public pre-K teachers and school-sponsored pre-K teachers fared better, at about $34,000 and $43,000, respectively. Kindergarten and elementary teachers earned about $53,000 and $56,000, respectively.

As a result, economic insecurity is a significant concern among those in the early care and education workforce, Whitebook said. Forty-six percent of child care workers participate in some kind of federal income support (e.g., the Earned Income Tax Credit, Medicaid, food stamps), and many receive state- or local-level subsidies (e.g., child care subsidies, housing support). Many also hold down second jobs. Whitebook mentioned a study from several years ago in which teachers were asked to rate what they worry about and their level of financial security through their job. The resulting data showed that those who were earning more were worrying less, which is not unexpected, Whitebook said. People with more education worry less than those who do not have as much education (which is likely related to earnings). However, a substantial portion of people with degrees were still worrying about their monthly bills and providing food for their own families, and the worry was greater for those with young children.

An important skill for teachers, Whitebook said, is the ability to have intentional interactions with children. This requires them to remain focused and present in the moment. Economic insecurity can cause significant stress and can distract teachers from focusing on children's needs. That stress, brought on by low pay and inadequate benefits, can be exacerbated by job conditions (many responsibilities, little down time, physical demands, etc.) and job instability. Whitebook mentioned the work of Megan Gunnar of the University of Minnesota, who has said that to be a good preschool teacher, one must have good executive function, but stress affects the areas of the brain and the capacities that teachers need to be most effective. Whitebook also referred participants to a study by

Whitaker and colleagues, which found that signs of poor physical and mental health occurred at a much higher rate among Head Start staff in Pennsylvania than among others in the United States with comparable sociodemographic characteristics (Whitaker et al., 2013).

In closing, Whitebook quoted the IOM and NRC workforce consensus report as saying that

> young children thrive when they have secure, positive relationships with adults who are knowledgeable about how to support their development and learning and are responsive to their individual progress. Thus, the adults who provide for their care and education bear a great responsibility. (IOM and NRC, 2015, p. 1)

Society in turn has a great responsibility to these early childhood teachers, of whom so much is expected, but to whom so little is given, Whitebook said. Maintaining and developing better health for children and families requires the expertise and the support of these professionals.

EMBEDDING SOCIAL-EMOTIONAL LEARNING INTO STATE POLICIES

Grafwallner began by pointing out that Brotman's discussion of ParentCorps and its emphasis on self-regulation, Askew's description of early childhood mental health consultation in New York City, and Whiteman's and LeMoine's overview of the workforce competencies needed to support children's healthy development all have one common topic—ensuring children's ability to have equitable access to SEL opportunities. The Council of Chief State School Officers (CCSSO) has been working with the Collaboration of Academic, Social, and Emotional Learning to incorporate aspects of SEL into schools and early childhood programs. Language in the Every Student Succeeds Act (ESSA) (the latest iteration of the Elementary and Secondary Education Act) provides an opportunity for a stronger emphasis on "soft skills" (i.e., SEL) to be incorporated into the ESSA plans, including into accountability plans. Over the last year, most of the chief state school officers have been focused on developing and implementing ESSA plans in their states.

Competencies of SEL

The competencies of SEL, Grafwallner said, include self-awareness (i.e., the identification of emotions and self-confidence); self-management skills (e.g., self-regulation, impulse control, self-motivation, goal setting, organizational skills); responsible decision making (making choices based on respect and empathy for others); relationship building (social engagement); and social awareness (identifying problems and being able to solve them) (for more information, see Gayl, 2017).

These competencies apply to early childhood education as well as to K–12. Interestingly, Grafwallner said, the research on these skills is extremely rich and robust for early childhood education, but there is a dearth of research on SEL in elementary and secondary education. A question that needs attention, he added, is how to sustain work on SEL competencies beyond early care and education and on through K–12.

ESSA Plans

ESSA calls for integrating SEL into "well-rounded education." Grafwallner discussed several aspects of the ESSA plans that CCSSO works on and provided examples of actions that states are taking.

How do states define well-rounded education in their plans? States define SEL skills to reflect children's need to understand and manage emotion, set goals, and build positive relationships. Illinois, for example, has established pre-K to grade 12 SEL standards, and the implementation of these standards is supported by integration into multi-tiered support systems (MTSSs) in public schools. Grafwallner said that five other states are also in the process of establishing standards.

How is SEL represented in the plans? States can provide professional development on SEL competencies. For example, Massachusetts is including sustained professional development for teachers and guidance to local school districts and schools on how they can incorporate SEL into their curricula.

How is SEL being implemented and operationalized? State education agencies have programs to support the behavioral needs of students, such as positive behavioral interventions and supports (PBISs), MTSSs, and wrap-around services. There is an emphasis on supporting students on all fronts, Grafwallner said. Delaware is working with low-performing schools in high-need communities to establish more comprehensive services for early childhood mental health support, with wrap-around services to sustain support through the primary grades.

Finally, how is SEL connected to the various issues related to accountability for schools? For the first time, ESSA has given states the opportunity to evaluate soft skills (i.e., not academic skills) to help identify low-performing schools and to also consider other areas that are very important to families and parents. State accountability systems may now include indicators of school quality, such as school climate or school discipline (e.g., suspensions). States are promoting alignment of early childhood mental health consultation with PBIS or MTSS for K–12. As an example, Iowa is establishing data systems to follow a variety of indicators (e.g., emotional safety conditions) using the Safe and Supportive Schools Condition for Learning Index. These states are trailblazers, working to sustain SEL across the board, Grafwallner concluded.

PARTNERING WITH THE BUSINESS COMMUNITY

There are many opportunities for collaboration to apply early childhood learning to improve public health. Higgins shared a figure from the 2014 roundtable workshop that illustrates potential health and development trajectories from early childhood to later life as well as the impacts of both stressors and interventions, including education, on a child's trajectory (see Figure 4-3). She emphasized the need to broaden the audience of individuals and organizations that participate in these collaborations and discussed the role of the business community. EPIC, she said, is a business advocacy organization that works to enlighten the business community, at the highest levels, to be aware of the importance of early childhood education, and get the community to engage.[3]

Employers, whether public, private, or government, are very motivated to support early childhood education, Higgins said, and she encouraged participants to engage with the business community and business leaders. There are some businesses that are very generous, philanthropic, and community-minded, she said. Most, however, have arrived at a position of "enlightened self-interest," realizing the impact that early childhood education has on the future availability of skilled employees. She noted that the millennial generation is entering the workforce, and she said that they have different commitments and needs from their employers. Another aspect that businesses have come to recognize is the costs due to employee child care challenges. Statistical analysis can estimate the costs of child care–related absenteeism, staff turnover, lost productivity, and inability to fill open job positions. In some cases, employers are willing to make a commitment to help support early care and education in a way that makes sense to them and their business.

There are other motivations for the business sector to become engaged in early care and education issues, Higgins said. In particular, there are tax-advantaged opportunities, such as tax credits or tax deductions, which are ways to share the cost of partnering to support early childhood education. Higgins offered these three examples:

1. **The Cafeteria Plan** (under Section 125 of the Internal Revenue Code) allows employees to choose from a menu of benefits to

[3] See http://www.coloradoepic.org (accessed October 30, 2017).

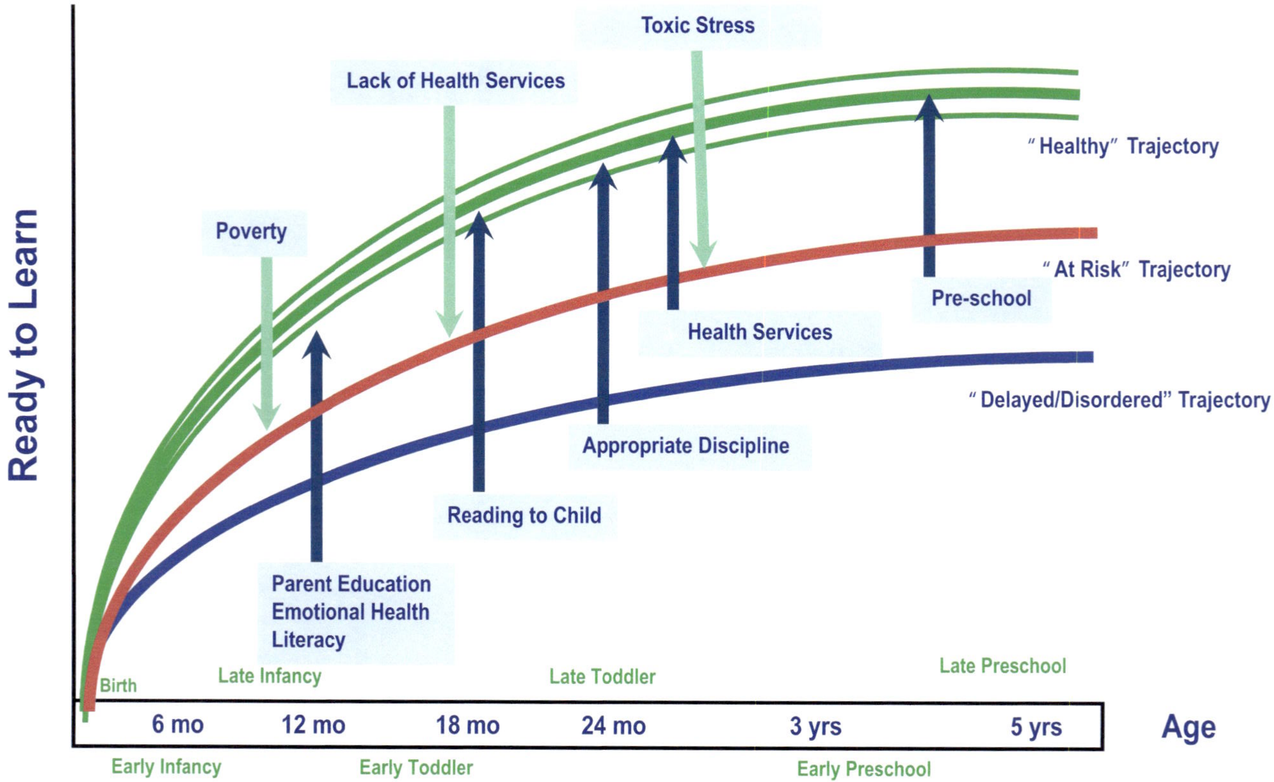

FIGURE 4-3 Opportunities for collaboration to influence health along the early childhood learning trajectory.
SOURCES: Higgins presentation, September 14, 2017, reprinted from IOM, 2015 (from the Halfon, 2014, presentation).

create a package that is best for their needs and to pay for those benefits with pre-tax income (e.g., health care, flexible spending accounts to pay child care expenses). This results in tax benefits for both employee and employer. Higgins said that these types of benefits can be very beneficial for the significant share of working-class individuals who could be defined as working class poor.

2. **Dependent Care Assistance Programs** (under Section 129 of the Internal Revenue Code) allow employers to contribute to an employee's child care cost through the Cafeteria Plan mechanism, up to $5,000 per year. The employee receives that benefit income tax free. Higgins noted that the total annual contribution for the child care flexible spending account is capped at $5,000, which dates back to a 1982 law. She is currently advocating that the cap be updated to adjust for inflation.
3. **The Colorado Child Care Contribution Tax Credit** (a Colorado statute) provides a 50 percent tax credit for qualified contributions to child care programs. For example, if an employer has many workers who use a particular child care center and the employer chooses to support that center, the employer will get a Colorado tax credit for half of what it donates.

EPIC advocates at the federal level and at the business level for family-friendly workplace policies, Higgins said. At the business level, the goal is to enlighten employers about ways they can support work–life balance for their employees by providing simple solutions at low cost to the employer. Such solutions might include flex time, job sharing, or perhaps combining funding sources (vacation time, sick time, disability insurance, corporate generosity) to maximize paid, or partially paid, maternity or paternity leave.

In conclusion, Higgins said, EPIC works to engage businesses and to allow them to use their voice, at the policy level and the workplace level, to make a difference for their employees.

HEALTH CARE AND CHILD CARE INTEGRATION

The Permanent Fund for Vermont's Children is the largest nonprofit organization for early childhood work in the state of Vermont, Richards said.[4] Vermont is a small state, with a population of about 626,000 and an annual state budget of $5 billion. About 6,100 babies are born each year. Vermont is very rural and has deep pockets of poverty. There are also areas of great diversity, Richards said, and 45 languages other than

[4] See http://www.permanentfund.org (accessed October 30, 2017).

English are spoken in the Burlington-area school district. The state is using its small size to its advantage, working to break down silos and grow partnerships.

When the Permanent Fund was founded in 2000, it worked on adult-to-child mentoring and small, early childhood grants. Over the years it became more sophisticated, and several years ago all of the diverse funding was pulled together into one collaborative. The intent was to use philanthropy as an agent for sustainable, permanent change, Richards said. The Permanent Fund chose the most ambitious, but achievable goal it could identify and established a deadline. That goal is high-quality, affordable early care and learning for all who need it in Vermont, and the deadline is 2025. The entire endowment is committed to achieving this goal by this date, she said, and then the Permanent Fund will "go out of business."

It is not possible to accomplish such a huge societal change without linking to health care, Richards said, and the Permanent Fund is working on integrating health care and child care. The health community in Vermont is moving to a fee-for-outcomes payment system and a focus on prevention. Most children are in some form of out-of-home care, and an accessible, high-quality, affordable system of care could provide both a safe environment for children and a huge population for primary prevention activities. This would also be a cost-effective, streamlined platform on which to co-administer other health services.

Stakeholders from all sectors in Vermont are coming together to discuss issues of importance for the state, such as caring for today's workforce, training tomorrow's workforce, curbing health care costs, the developmental origins of health and disease, opioid abuse, and resiliency. Brain science has shown that significant brain architecture is built early in a child's life. The return on investment from early childhood development interventions is clear. And yet, Richards lamented, the pattern of actual spending is exactly opposite to the return on investment—in Vermont and everywhere else. In Vermont the public investment per child for infants and toddlers (age 0 to 2 years) is $903; for preschoolers (age 3 to 5 years) is $3,578; and for school-aged children (6 to 19 years) is $18,000.

The logical conclusion from this reality is simple: invest now or pay more later. A supply-and-demand analysis revealed that seven out of ten children under age 6 in Vermont have all available parents in the labor force, which means that they are likely to need some form of child care while a parent is working. Of these children likely to need child care, 47 percent of infants and toddlers do not have access to regulated child care, and 70 percent do not have access to high-quality, regulated child care. Furthermore, Richards said, child care is not affordable. The cost of child care, without subsidy, accounts for 40 percent of the gross household income of a single parent at median income.

The approach to tackling these issues includes public awareness, policy, and research and development innovation incubators, Richards said. She briefly described several initiatives the Permanent Fund is working on, including Vermont Birth to Five, which is focused on strengthening quality and systems, and the Let's Grow Kids public awareness campaign. One example of linking health care to child care is work the Permanent Fund has done with the health care system to have the medical community train child care providers to conduct developmental screens and referrals. They have blanketed the entire state, and child care providers in every region of the state have now been trained, she said. In addition, trust and communication have been built between these sectors.

CHANGING INSTITUTIONS AND THEIR CULTURES

At its core, improving population health by leveraging early childhood care and education is about institutional change and about changing institutional cultures, Ewen said. Everyone in attendance is all working at the intersection of early care and education and health, she continued. Regardless of position or title or program, people working in early childhood education should be considering health to improve outcomes for children, and people working in health should be considering early childhood education to improve outcomes for children. Everyone is a potential partner in this work. Child care providers, schools, pediatricians, family practitioners, community health workers, trainers and those in workforce development, workers in welfare offices, and those working on domestic violence, bullying prevention, and gun violence prevention are all part of the conversation about early care and education and health. There are roles for the public, policy makers, political leaders, and the private sector (business community, foundations). The philanthropic community, for example, can lead the way by funding data collection, pilot programs, communication strategies, and advocacy activities.

Ultimately, this issue is about assuring equity for children, Ewen said. Assuring equity for early care and education providers is also a core principle. Ewen emphasized that all voices are relevant and have a role in these collaborative conversations, from the executive directors of the largest organizations to the family child care providers serving children and families with special needs. It is also time, she said, to think differently about what outcomes matter at the intersection of early care and education and health. Efforts to close the achievement gap have long focused on language and math skills, but the achievement gap also stems from health and developmental factors.

Ewen offered several examples of changing policy and practice at the intersection of early care and education and health, which she presented in two categories: the intentional creation of new programs, practices, and policies; and seizing opportunities to "get on the train that is leaving the station."

Intentional Creation of New Programs, Practices, and Policies

Intentionality, Ewen said, is building a system, putting the pieces children need into it, and then seeing what happens. One example of intentionality is the universal pre-K program in New York City. A key component of the Pre-K for All program was building developmental screenings of all children into the program design. Early care providers have the resources and training to conduct developmental screenings. There is a process for tracking screenings, and there are now several years' worth of data available. The data show an increase in children being referred for supports and early intervention and also some specific health outcomes, including a significant decrease in asthma among young children. Asthma, Ewen noted, keeps a large number of children out of school. If these children can be identified and given the medical resources they need, they can stay in school and have a better chance at success. Head Start (discussed by Shinn-Brown in Chapter 3) and the SEL standards required by ESSA (discussed by Grafwallner) are other examples of intentionally creating new programs, practices, or policies that bring health and early education together.

Get on the Train That Is Leaving the Station

Good advocates often find ways to incorporate their issue into existing initiatives, Ewen said. Many communities are very invested in data collection. One example is the Early Development Instrument to measure school readiness (mentioned by Groginsky in Chapter 3), which is being implemented in a number of communities around the country. How can the volumes of data being collected be used to understand which children have access to high-quality early care and education in a community, where the family support programs are in that community, or where the pediatricians are in that community? How can these data be leveraged to create a community that is more supportive of children and families?

There are many opportunities to get on the train, Ewen said. Many communities, for example, have funders that want to build playgrounds, but if nobody uses them, they are of little value. There is an opportunity when those resources are being planned and built to bring policy makers together to make sure that children will be able to use them. In every state, children with disabilities who are in school systems are being assessed on a series of outcome measures. In many school districts and programs that are serving young children with disabilities (infants, toddlers, preschoolers), those outcome measures are only looked at for that population. How can those policy levers be pushed to expand those outcome measures to all children and their families? The Head Start program is required to conduct developmental and other screenings (e.g., hearing, vision). Often those screenings are donated. How can those screenings be provided to all children before they enter kindergarten?

Ewen concluded by emphasizing that a small group of people can come together around a common goal and make a big change in public perceptions. The DC Public Libraries had heard about the word gap research and saw an opportunity to use some of their public service money to educate families about how communicating with their children builds their vocabulary. They launched a public awareness campaign, and now, for example, people riding in a taxi cab in Washington, DC, will hear a public service announcement about Sing, Talk, and Read. Ewen encouraged participants to make sure that every action they take is about bringing early care and education and health together.

DISCUSSION

During the open discussion that followed the panel presentations, participants discussed the cost of providing high-quality care, from economic analyses and funding to the training and compensation of staff. Participants were particularly interested in the forthcoming National Academies consensus study on financing early care and education with a highly qualified workforce (mentioned by Whitebook, earlier). There was also interest in further information about the tax credits for businesses discussed by Higgins.

Paying for Quality

Kindig asked about any economic analyses in the early care and education sector that might help identify targets and whether excess spending in health care might be reallocated to meet some of the needs. Ewen responded that there are cost analyses of, for example, child care, universal child care, and universal paid leave. The costs of pre-K programs for all 3- and 4-year olds have been analyzed in DC and New York—the figures are large, and there are tradeoffs. She observed that there are many cultural and political reasons why people do not want to invest large sums of money in early childhood care and education. And even if additional investment in Medicaid does not increase affordable child care, it is worthwhile because it can be used to create preventive systems that serve mother and baby together. She emphasized the need for universal child care in the United States, arguing that child care should be considered a public good, similar to K–12 education, and should be paid for in the same way. Richards added that one way to move a huge public policy issue forward is to have a public body talk about it. The Vermont legislature established the Blue-Ribbon Commission on Financing High-Quality, Affordable Care, which over a period of 1.5 years held public discussions on the costs of providing high-quality early care for those who need it. They concluded that an additional $206 million per year would be needed to provide high-quality care for the 70 percent of the population likely to need care. That might sound small, she said, but for a state with a $5 billion budget, it is significant. The numbers and details are needed for advocacy efforts, she said.

Participants discussed the ongoing National Academies study on the cost of high-quality early care and education. Helene Stebbins of the Alliance for Early Success said that it will be important for advocates to get together in preparation for the release of the report in order to begin to gather support for and take action on the findings and recommendations. Richards emphasized the importance of working with the business community, adding that it is easier to justify public investment if it can be demonstrated that the private and philanthropic sectors are already doing their parts. She also spoke of the need for shared services and creating economies of scale around the micro units of child care providers in order to demonstrate efficiency to legislatures when seeking money. Finally, she said, it is very effective to explain that 100 percent of this money goes to people; it is not just for buying things. Jones agreed and said that the National Academies study is based on the notion that high-quality care is provided by well prepared, well trained, well compensated teachers. The cost of quality is due to the cost of having teachers with appropriate compensation and appropriate skills. Others agreed with the need to be prepared for the release of the report and to create momentum concerning the recommendations. Jones said that perhaps that is a charge for the workshop participants.

Marthe Gold asked about the level of training needed and the salaries required to ensure a high-quality workforce for early care and education. Jones, who was a member of the National Academies consensus committee on transforming the workforce, said that a well-prepared workforce would have a wide range of competencies related to child development, partnering with parents and other professionals, and other skills and might perhaps require a bachelor's degree or higher. She noted that the Boston Public Schools preschool program requires teachers to have a master's degree. The field must reach the point where it is acknowledged that this work is real, that training is required, and that compensation must be appropriate. Ewen emphasized that there will be a wide range of skills, all of which are professional. Someone caring for infants, for example, needs different skills, not fewer skills, than someone caring for 4-, 5-, or 6-year-olds.

Tax Credits

In response to a question, Higgins provided more details about the tax credits in Colorado. The tax credit has existed for nearly 20 years and is up for reauthorization again in 2018. Businesses are taking advantage of the credit, although the details of this are difficult to assess definitively as about 80 percent of businesses are small businesses that file their tax returns as partnerships. The Department of Revenue cannot identify the difference between an individual and a partnership because the cash flows through the business entity to the individual. About $50 million per year has been contributed to child care centers, which is a meaningful amount of money, she said. The money is very broadly used. For example, it can be used to open a new child care center, to pay salaries, to pay for scholarships for families, or to pay for scholarships for the workforce. Colorado has tried to pass tax increases that would benefit early childhood education, but taxpayers have not been willing to entrust the spending of their dollars to the state legislature.

GALLERY WALK REFLECTIONS

Participants were presented with four questions in the final gallery walk.

1. What are the main policy levers that could support the spread and scale of health/early care and education coordination?
2. What does it mean to be ready for spread and scale, conceptually and practically? Or, what are guiding principles for jurisdictions deciding how to support early care and education/health connections?
3. How can policy create incentives for cross-sector collaboration?
4. Can you offer any new insights?

After everyone had reconvened, Lantz summarized individual participants' responses to the questions posed in the gallery and moderated the discussion. She recalled the point made by Whitebook that the way child care is set up in the United States is misaligned with what is well-understood about child development. Child care in the United States is, for the most part, a private market, and most people pay out of pocket for early care and education. The subsidies that are available are not reaching all of those who need them. The market also pays a very low wage to its workers. This system reinforces and exacerbates inequalities for children and creates psychosocial and financial stress for families and caregivers.

As a demographer, Lantz observed that the U.S. system is not pronatalist in its support of families as are many other countries around the world. The number of women giving birth has declined, and fertility rates are lower. Rates differ according to socioeconomic status. In many countries, women with higher levels of education are not having as many babies. A country's policies on support for families and young children affect birth rates, especially for women who are in the labor force. When countries have lower rates of reproduction, it alters the dependency ratio, which is the ratio of the number of children and older people (the dependent population) to the working-age population. Arguments about the need to invest more in children often seem to fall on deaf ears, Lantz said, or do not motivate the needed investments. In many countries, what has motivated policy makers to take more policy action in support of families and children has been the realization that there might not be enough children being born to support the population as its ages.

In reflecting on the comments that were made in the gallery, Lantz highlighted several main topic areas:

- **Partnerships.** Many of the comments posted called for investing in initiating and strengthening partnerships and collaborative approaches among the early care and education sector, the health sector, businesses, government, criminal justice, community organizers, and community members, to make the case for why more investments are needed and to develop specific plans. Lantz reported that one comment suggested looking to tobacco control and obesity prevention for successes from these kinds of partnerships and collaborations that could serve as models.
- **Special issues and insights.** Comments posted raised a range of topics and questions that had not yet been discussed at the workshop, including whether there is a role for respectful family planning to help women better plan, time, and space their pregnancies. Investments in this area might have positive impacts in terms of early childhood outcomes. Other topics raised included special issues for children in foster care, the impact of sleep on early childhood and development, and the impact of school absenteeism, Lantz reported. There were also comments about the community benefit investments required of nonprofit hospitals, including suggestions that early care and education be considered in every community health needs assessment.

- **Social impact bonds.** Lantz suggested that social impact bonds (pay-for-success financing) could be used to spread and scale interventions that would have a positive impact on early childhood development and population health. Chicago, for example, has a social impact bond initiative where private funders are investing in a pilot test of high-quality pre-K. The program is being evaluated, and the investors are receiving payments when success milestones are met.

Sources of Funding

During the discussion, a participant pointed out that South Carolina has a social impact bond for the Nurse–Family Partnership home visiting program and suggested that development issues, such as closing the word gap thorough talking and reading to children, could be incorporated into the visits. Robert McLellan of the Dartmouth-Hitchcock Medical Center pointed out that engaging private investors has been helpful in driving energy conservation and environmental sustainability efforts, as investors saw better returns from investing in energy efficiency than other marketplace efforts. Lantz suggested that there is a parallel between that example and social impact bond projects.

Following up on the point about hospital community benefit investments, Mary Pittman of the Public Health Institute said that much more money goes into the community from banks through the Community Development Fund. There are examples of investments in housing and transportation centers that have also had some linkage to education. She suggested exploring whether early care and education investment strategies could be incorporated into new initiatives from this fund.

Terry Allan of the Cuyahoga County Board of Health pointed out that some of the income from the Philadelphia sugar-sweetened-beverage tax is used to fund early childhood development and education programs. He noted that a similar tax initiative in Ohio in the late 1990s failed at the state level because the income was designated to go into the state general fund and was not tied to a specific use. Use taxes tied to a specific use, where there is a demonstrated need, appear to be more successful.

Chang said there is great potential for innovative funding in this area. She suggested, for example, urging the Center for Medicare & Medicaid Innovation to focus on children's health.

Sustainability of Funding

Ewen said that piecemeal approaches will not secure the funding needed. About 15 states have done economic impact studies of how much child care contributes to their state economy. In California, for example, child care is the third-largest generator of income to the state, after agriculture and tourism. Still, there have not been significant funding increases from the public sector in early childhood programs. The return on investment for early childhood investments ranges from $6 to $52 per $1 spent, depending on the study. She emphasized that sustainable approaches to funding are needed. During the last election cycle, for example, Ohio had passed a tax proposal to create 4-year-old pre-K programs. Although this is a great first step, she said, it is not clear if it will be sustainable (e.g., if it will need to be voted on periodically, or if it can be overturned). Various innovative and sustainable funding approaches are needed, including putting early childhood programs in school funding formulas and ensuring that tax policies pay for high-quality early care and education at the time when families need it. Lantz added that pay-for-success or social impact bonds are generally a proof-of-concept approach and are not themselves sustainable. The potential of the model is to fund innovative programs with private investor dollars to demonstrate to the government that a program or intervention is effective, at which point then government would assume financial responsibility for implementing such a program or intervention.

5

Closing Remarks and Reflections on the Day

In the final session of the workshop, George Isham, a roundtable co-chair, and Phyllis Meadows, a senior fellow in the health program at the Kresge Foundation, reflected on the workshop presentations and discussions and called upon roundtable members and participants to share their final observations.

Reflecting on Lantz's point about the perils of an altered dependency ratio (see Chapter 4), Isham observed that the older generation might not necessarily see the benefit of some of the policy changes concerning early care and education. At the other end of the spectrum, children's advocates often assume that children's welfare itself is sufficient justification for investments in early care and education. There is a need to look beyond the short-term outcomes and develop a rationale that is persuasive to other segments in society. There is a two-way learning curve involved in making an effective case for broader investment in early care and education in order to win supporting votes from across a wide spectrum of the country.

Isham also suggested that the tax incentives discussed by Higgins (see Chapter 4) have much broader applications for funding population health improvement policies and initiatives beyond early childhood. He suggested that the roundtable continue to pursue those avenues.

A one-size policy package does not fit all, Isham said, and it will be important to more fully understand the individual needs of states and regions across the country and also their policy environments (e.g., what works best for motivating local decision makers to support the type of early childhood strategies discussed at the workshop). Collaboration is needed across geography, as well as across sectors.

Meadows reflected on the notion of policy and practice intersection across sectors, what it really means, and what it will deliver on behalf of children and families. She highlighted several themes from the workshop discussions that were in line with the strategic direction of the health team at The Kresge Foundation:

- **Defining outcomes.** There is a broad range of outcomes that can be achieved at the intersection of early care and education and health. Sometimes, in trying to achieve so much, people in the field end up doing very little, Meadows said. She highlighted the need to be clear about the outcomes that the sectors are trying to achieve together.
- **Unleashing capital.** Kresge is working to unleash investments from anchor institutions, businesses, and other sectors and to identify new ways of financing programs that are important for the health of children and families.
- **Funding and policy challenges.** There was discussion about funding challenges and policy challenges. Meadows said that there are existing activities that could be leveraged for benefiting early care and education. For example, the community benefit activities conducted by nonprofit hospitals are already exploring population health and thinking about upstream activities needed.
- **Communities can define the solutions.** Strategically, Kresge is operating under the assumption that communities can define the solutions, Meadows said. This includes people who represent the community through their work every day, as many of the workshop participants do. Listening more closely to the community will help ensure that the foundation is making investments that will have meaning for the community, she said. Cross-sector collaborations are hard, she acknowledged, and communities that are already struggling are now being asked to participate in this collaboration. Those who have the resources, the research, and the body of talent need to determine how to be more supportive in forging these collaborative relationships. The need for leadership spans every dimension of the work discussed.

One of the goals of the roundtable is to think about how to take the best ideas and support the field in turning them into reality, Meadows said, and she shared her list of additional themes and ideas that stood out to her. First, she said, in this situation it is important to start both small and big. Leadership goes beyond training, she continued, and includes developing leaders as advocates. The early childhood workforce is at the center of bridging equity for children, but the burden should not be on those workers alone. There are many others who could offset the burden and augment the work that early care providers are doing.

One point of intersection where both early childhood providers and health providers focus is prevention. In serving children from age 0 to 5, both sectors are seeing the impacts of poor housing, poverty, safety concerns, lack of food, and trauma on both education and health outcomes. Another point of intersection is that these children and families are struggling in their interactions with the system. There are system failures and policy failures in both the educational system and the health system that are affecting the most vulnerable children, Meadows said.

In an optimistic vein, Meadows posed several questions for thought. What would it look like if all children (regardless of race, social and economic status, or geography) had available, affordable, relevant access to the services they need to be healthy, to thrive, and to learn? What if all states were moving aggressively toward safe, affordable care, like Vermont, or created streamlined platforms to ensure that health is connected to early childhood care and learning, like Nemours? What if all of the workshop participants walked away embracing the idea that they are all working at the intersection of early care and education and health? What if the early care and education and health systems were so aligned and connected that children were experiencing the best possible outcomes that they could?

DISCUSSION

Making the Case for Children

Robert McLellan of Dartmouth Hitchcock suggested that there is a need to bring communication science to these issues. He described the challenges of convincing decision makers of a need for action, even when armed with robust evidence of a problem. Those working in the population health field need to learn how to talk to the right people, in the right language, and frame the conversation in a way that will bring results. For example, he noted the difference between having an equity conversation and an opportunity conversation with decision makers. Philip Alberti of the Association of American Medical Colleges suggested that a real focus on community engagement and partnership has been missing from the conversation. It is necessary to understand the outcomes and metrics that matter to funders, philanthropists, teachers, school board members, and whoever else in the community must be convinced to support funding. Understanding which arguments will garner support comes through conversations and engagement with the community. Alberti agreed with Isham on the importance of understanding state-by-state policies, frameworks, and legislatures. He raised concerns about issues of racism, classism, and xenophobia that give rise to the inequities that can lead to the childhood and adult outcomes that have not been successfully addressed. He emphasized the need to engage all sectors of society in meaningful, bi-directional partnerships and to understand the metrics that matter to those sectors of society.

Meadows wondered aloud, "What if every state were like Vermont?" Richards responded that Vermont does not have it all figured out, listing some of the challenges on the path to improving outcomes. The state, she added, is struggling with the crisis of the affordability, quality, and outcomes of early childhood education as well as with various socioeconomic issues. There are deep pockets of poverty throughout the entire state and children who are at risk for a range of concerns. What can be learned from Vermont and potentially replicated elsewhere, Richards said, is the staging of a successful campaign and advocacy effort. She agreed that there is a need to identify the outcome—or several outcomes—that link the early care and education and the health sectors together, adding that the sectors can then coalesce around those priority issues and start building momentum together.

Fostering Cross-Sector Dialogue

Higgins added a question to Meadows's generative list, asking, What if the health care industry took the leadership, and invited the early childhood community to come in and address it as subject-matter experts? If the health care community endorsed early care and education and its importance to public health and population health, it could totally change the dialogue, she said. Isham agreed and said that a dialogue between the sectors needs to draw first upon the expertise in each sector to educate the other about the options and possibilities.

Marthe Gold of The New York Academy of Medicine suggested that if the roundtable were to broaden its agenda by changing its title to a Roundtable on Population Well-Being, it would have a greater ability to bring in people from a broader range of sectors and enlarge the circles of conversations and understanding.

Funding and Sustainability

Chang reflected on the allocation of resources and emphasized political will as a key program accelerator, along with champions and leadership. She reiterated the need for sustainability, both financial and with respect to how programs are implemented, so that they are embedded into the fabric of current existing programs and involve community capacity building.

Adding to Meadows's list of questions for thought, Mary Pittman asked, What if there was a way to connect all the services that the families need in addition to early childhood education? What if funds from the Special Supplemental Nutrition Program for Women, Infants, and Children; Medicaid; food stamps; and tax incentives could be braided to create a pool of funds that is set aside to ensure that all of the lowest-income families have free access? She suggested a pilot program to gauge interest, pulling those dollars together to provide vouchers to the lowest-income families.

Specific Vulnerable Populations

Pamela Russo said that there is still a considerable need to address lead exposure in children, and she suggested incorporating this into partnerships between public health and early childhood. Chang also raised the issue of those children in family child care, who are among the most vulnerable children.

A

References

Bureau of Children, Youth, and Families, New York City Department of Health and Mental Hygiene. 2017. Public Health Approach to Early Childhood Mental Health. Presented by George Askew at the Roundtable on Population Health Improvement's workshop Exploring Early Childhood Care and Education Levers to Improve Population Health, New York, NY.

Campbell F., G. Conti, J. J. Heckman, S. H. Moon, R. Pinto, E. Pungello, and Y. Pan. 2014. Early childhood investments substantially boost adult health. *Science* 343(6178):1478–1485.

Gayl, C. L. 2017. *How state planning for the every student succeeds act (ESSA) can promote student academic, social, and emotional learning: An examination of five key strategies.* Collaborative for Academic, Social, and Emotional Learning. http://www.casel.org/wp-content/uploads/2017/04/ESSA-and-SEL-Five-Strategies-April-2017-041717.pdf (accessed May 10, 2018).

Hart, B., and T. R. Risley. 1995. *Meaningful differences in the everyday experience of young American children.* Baltimore, MD: Paul H. Brookes Publishing Company.

IOM (Institute of Medicine). 2015. *Exploring opportunities for collaboration between health and education to improve population health: Workshop summary.* Washington, DC: The National Academies Press. doi: https://doi.org/10.17226/18979.

IOM and NRC (National Research Council). 2015. *Transforming the workforce for children birth through age 8: A unifying foundation.* Washington, DC: The National Academies Press. doi: https://doi.org/10.17226/19401.

Jacobson, D., and S. Teutsch. 2012. An environmental scan of integrated approaches for defining and measuring total population health by the clinical care system, the government public health system, and stakeholder organizations. Commissioned Paper. http://www.improvingpopulationhealth.org/PopHealthPhaseIICommissionedPaper.pdf (accessed May 10, 2018).

Kindig, D., and G. Stoddart. 2003. What is population health? *American Journal of Public Health* 93(3):380–383.

Klass, P., B. P. Dreyer, and A. L. Mendelsohn. 2009. Reach out and read: Literacy promotion in pediatric primary care. *Advamces in Pediatrics* 56:11–27.

NASEM (National Academies of Sciences, Engineering, and Medicine). 2017. *Communities in action: Pathways to health equity*. Washington, DC: The National Academies Press. doi: https://doi.org/10.17226/24624.

Thompson, R. A., and C. A. Nelson. 2001. Developmental science and the media: Early brain development. *American Psychologist* 56(1):5–15.

Whitaker, R. C., B. D. Becker, A. N. Herman, and R. A. Gooze. 2013. The physical and mental health of Head Start staff: The Pennsylvania Head Start Staff Wellness Survey, 2012. *Preventing Chronic Disease* 10:E181.

Whitebook, M., D. Phillips, and C. Howes. 2014. *Worthy work, STILL unlivable wages: The early childhood workforce 25 years after the National Child Care Staffing Study*. Berkeley, CA: Center for the Study of Child Care Employment, University of California, Berkeley.

B

Workshop Agenda

Early Childhood Care and Education Levers to
Improve Population Health
September 14, 2017

Location: Farkas Auditorium,
New York University Langone Medical Center,
550 First Avenue, New York City

WORKSHOP OBJECTIVES

The workshop is intended to explore in as much depth as possible the intersection of health and early care and education—with attention to equity, birth through age 5, and across all early care and education settings—in order to surface and understand potential effects on population health. Presentations and discussion are intended to

1. highlight what is working at the intersection of health and early care and education, discuss the importance of early care and education in achieving overall goals for early childhood development, and consider current priorities;
2. provide examples of successful initiatives focused on early care and education and health; and
3. create space for conversations around the examples provided, including spread and scale for greater impact, sustainability

(including funding models), the collection of relevant data, and the identification of additional gaps that need to be addressed.

8:30 a.m. **Welcome and opening remarks**

George Isham, senior advisor, HealthPartners, senior fellow, HealthPartners Institute for Education and Research; co-chair, Roundtable on Population Health Improvement

8:45 a.m. **Workshop purpose and overview**

Debbie Chang, senior vice president, Policy and Prevention, Nemours; member, planning committee; member, Roundtable on Population Health Improvement; and Phyllis Meadows, senior fellow, Health Program, The Kresge Foundation; member, planning committee; member, Roundtable on Population Health Improvement

9:00 a.m. **TOPIC 1: THE EVIDENCE—exploring what works in early childhood care in areas (evidence for policy along with evidence for programs, practices, and implementation) that health sector partners can support, including advocating for evidence-based policies and programs**

Moderator: *Danielle Ewen, senior policy advisor, EducationCounsel, LLC*

Speaker: *Judith Carta, interim director, Juniper Gardens Children's Project; senior scientist, Institute for Life Span Studies; professor, Special Education, University of Kansas*

Discussants:

Laurie Brotman, Bezos Family Foundation Professor of Early Childhood Development, Department of Population Health, New York University

Alison Gertel-Rosenberg, director, National Prevention and Practice, Nemours

Jodi Whiteman, director of professional development, Zero to Three

Sarah LeMoine, director, Early Childhood Workforce Innovations, Zero to Three

9:45 a.m. **Q&A**

Moderator: *Danielle Ewen*

10:00 a.m. **Break**

10:15 a.m. **Topic 1 Gallery Walk**

Moderator: *Valora Washington, chief executive officer, Council for Professional Recognition*

Questions

a. How can the field better apply what is known at interface of early care and education and health (e.g., screening for developmental milestones)?
b. What are the gaps and white spaces that need to be prioritized?
c. What are the new insights (e.g., what you need to know about parents, teachers, caregivers)

10:50 a.m. **Reporting back from Topic 1 gallery walk**

Moderator: *Valora Washington*

11:10 a.m. **TOPIC 2: CROSS-SECTOR COLLABORATION (examples and lessons)**

Moderator: *Debbie Chang*

Speaker: *George Askew, deputy commissioner, New York City Department of Health and Mental Hygiene Division of Family and Child Health*

Discussants:

Kimberly Shinn-Brown, program director, Ozarks Area Community Action Corporation Head Start/Early Head Start, Springfield, Missouri

Krista Scott, senior director of health policy, Child Care Aware

Michelle Suarez, early childhood developer, Prosper Lincoln, Nebraska Children and Families Foundation

12:05 p.m. **Q&A**

Moderator: *Debbie Chang*

12:20 p.m. **LUNCH** (provided for members and speakers; neighborhood options available to attendees at registration desk)

1:20 p.m. **Topic 2 Gallery Walk**

Moderator: *Larry Pasti, senior director, Big Picture Approach Consulting, Forum for Youth Investing*

Questions

a. How can we accelerate cross-sectoral collaboration in early care education and health? What do you need to help you and your organization collaborate effectively?
b. What are the main barriers to collaboration and the solutions to them?
c. What have we learned from other cross-sector collaborations that could help to inform early care and education/health interactions?
d. What are the new insights?

2:00 p.m. **Reporting back from Topic 2 gallery walk**

Moderator: *Larry Pasti*

2:20 p.m. **Break**

2:30 p.m. **TOPIC 3: Policy challenges and opportunities at the intersection of early care and education and health (i.e., questions of finance, workforce, equity)**

Moderator: *Jacqueline Jones, president and chief executive officer, Foundation for Child Development*

Speaker: *Marcy Whitebook, director, Center for Study of Child Care Employment, University of California, Berkeley*

Discussants:
Rolf Grafwallner, program director for early childhood initiatives, Council of Chief State School Officers
Gloria Higgins, executive director, Executives Partnering to Invest in Children
Aly Richards, chief executive officer, The Permanent Fund for Vermont's Children
Danielle Ewen

3:35 p.m. **Q&A**

Moderator: *Jacqueline Jones*

3:50 p.m. **Topic 3 Gallery Walk**

Moderator: *Paula Lantz, associate dean for Academic Affairs, professor of public policy, Gerald R. Ford School of Public Policy, University of Michigan*

Questions

a. What are the priority interventions and policies related to early childhood care and education that should be spread and scaled?
b. What policy actions can be taken to address some of the challenges in spreading and scaling effective early childhood care and education interventions and programs?
c. What needs to be done to support and increase investments for new ideas and innovation in early childhood care and education?
d. What policy actions can be taken to increase collaboration and synergies between those working in the health sector and the early childhood care and education sector?

4:20 p.m. **Reporting back from Topic 3 gallery walk**

Moderator: *Paula Lantz*

4:35 p.m. **Closing remarks and reflections on the day**
Phyllis Meadows
George Isham

5:00 p.m. **Adjourn**

Thank you to the planning committee and to all invited guests, both presenters and those in the audience, including Elizabeth Groginsky (DC Office of the State Superintendent of Education), Cody Kornack (National Head Start Association), Nancy Lim (National League of Cities), and Bridget Walsh (Schuyler Center for Analysis and Advocacy).

C

Gallery Walk Questions and Input

ACRONYMS AND ABBREVIATIONS IN THE GALLERY WALK COMMENTS

ACO	accountable care organization
CHNA	Community Health Needs Assessments
CMMI	Center for Medicare & Medicaid Innovation
ECE	early childhood education
EMR	electronic medical record
FOA	Funding Opportunity Announcement
IRS	Internal Revenue Service
MACRA	Medicare Access and CHIP [Children's Health Insurance Program] Reauthorization Act of 2015
MCH	maternal and child health
MIPS	merit-based incentive payments system
National Academies	National Academies of Sciences, Engineering, and Medicine
NYC	New York City

OB obstetrician

PED pediatrician

ROI return on investment

Topic 1: Evidence

a. How can the field better apply what is known at the interface of ECE and health (e.g., screening for developmental milestones)?
   - Monthly happy birthday–type materials sent to families with information on milestones and low- to no-cost ways to help child develop.
   - Better data collection in child care, better use of data to target resources to underserved populations.
   - Business leaders and health administrator awareness and commitment to investments and ROI of ECE.
   - Create community demand.
   - Public awareness for all community sectors is critical.
   - Discharge moms/babies from hospitals with materials that promote talking/singing to infants.
   - Create health teams that include personnel trained in developmental screening and deploy community health workers to do home visits regarding books/songs at home.
   - Define a lean/minimal set of outcome measures at key milestones.
   - Focus on concrete, doable actions at each level and with community, state, and regional leaders to share messages and lessons learned and *why* it matters—so what? What's in it for me?
   - Share those effective cross-sector partnerships that are sustainable.
   - Compatible software systems that enable more providers to access records and ability to share information.
   - Consider social genome[1] indicators in longitudinal follow-up.
   - Shift the dialogue to assure promotion of developmental health and healthy relationships (primary prevention).
   - Important to have awareness of predictive risk for developmental delays (e.g., income, adverse childhood experiences) and ensure services (parent support, home visiting, early literacy, implemented at population level).
   - How does ECE fit into the logic model leading to longer, better quality of life and better distribution (more equitable) of those outcomes in the population?

[1] See http://www.social-genome.org (accessed May 15, 2018).

- More support of systems-level integration of ECE into pediatric settings.
- Don't be fixated on obesity as a "health" outcome. Social, emotional, mental health, and academic outcomes are a pathway for better lifetime health broadly conceived (as opposed to one narrow outcome).
- Promote more exemplars—tell the story with more than stats.
- How can the power of health care advance the goals of ECE—which will improve health?
- How to connect this work to third-grade reading and other initiatives (e.g., social-emotional learning in schools and community) for support longitudinally.
- Familial screening regarding social, psychological, and behavioral factors that influence education and health, and the collection of screening findings in EMR.
- Necessity of creating a shared language across public health, medical field, and education fields to talk about shared desirable outcomes.
- Remember opportunity for bidirectional connections between ECE and pediatric care (e.g., ECE as setting to advance health).
- Health care (pediatrics) as a platform for promoting child development.
- Look to local level for solutions.
- Top down doesn't work.
- It is in the details that the solutions are found.
- De-jargoning terms, creating better engagement for providers in professional development, language access, cultural norms, opportunities/time for professional development.
- Invest in consultant models in child care (mental health, child care, health consultants).
- We have to talk about financing more!
- We know many things to be done; we need to prioritize funding and work with policy makers on creative options (e.g., social impact bonds).
- Screening and referral and follow-up to ensure service delivery is available for early childhood medical homes.
- Need examples of best practices that go step by step—funding sources, partners, how to make evidence actionable.
- Using/encouraging longitudinal data systems that integrate health and education data to identify which best practices are most scalable and for whom these practices work best.
- Funding could be attached to partnering across disciplines to look for innovations.

- Bi-directional communication.
- Not only data, but terminology and goals.

b. What are the gaps and white spaces that need to be prioritized?
- How to develop an infrastructure of trainers and coaches to deliver evidence-based training to care providers from birth to age 3.
- Funding.
- Family-based child care, systemic support, training and learning collaboratives for this group.
- Raising salaries and ECE training/professional education for providers.
- How the relationships between parenting and child outcomes vary by culture.
- Need more evidence on quality-improvement approach in ECE integration work.
- Impact of the health, safety, and well-being of ECE personal on ECE outcomes.
- How to reach the informal day care providers, early childhood care given in their homes.
- How does the Head Start experience fit?
- Need to consider the social environmental facts that impact the well-being of children.
- Child poverty is a factor—how is the ECE sector engaging to address the issue for families?
- Effective communication with families and teachers and health care providers. How is information shared with parents? Are parents able to reinforce learning and advocate for their child's needs? How do non-regular work schedules for parent's impact ability to connect with/communicate with providers?
- What is the relative balance of inputs to child development outcomes: word gap, nutrition, parent education, etc., and the relative investment benchmark of each (i.e., per capita $)?
- Family violence prevention and healthy relationships.
- How do you get this type of thinking infusion in higher education for the next generation of professionals?
- Child outcomes with disparity breakouts.
- Are optimal ECE programs including trauma-informed care?
- What efforts are under way to address the "hand-off" process from early childhood to future life-stage work?
- Who is an ECE provider? Is a home visitor? Is an early intervention provider?

- Research and evidence-based programs are emerging that create the opportunity to take them to scale; the challenge that we face is to honor diversity, family income, and rural versus urban settings.
- Do public awareness campaigns around the word gap work? What is the evidence?
- Addressing the social determinants of health of children and families.
- Providing a full assessment to ensure children/families are getting the appropriate services.
- We have better common understanding that outcomes are much more than reading and math. How do we convey this better, more widely, across sectors?
- How to identify children who are beginning to show language delays before they are officially eligible for early intervention services (Part C).
- Bridge between academic and education systems.
- Gain clarity that sectors that touch families in first 1,000 days—home visiting, parent support, early intervention, primary care (OB/PED)—are clearly defined as part of early care system.
- Is there policy agreement on child development outcomes . . . overall and at each age stage?
- Collaboration—how do you support local collaboration, [it is] not in the budgets of the different stakeholders.
- How best should these diverse approaches be synthesized or jointly implemented to minimize redundancy and maximize impact?
- Support for infrastructure that promotes collaboration: shared metrics, time for providers, leaders, and parents to align and coordinate toward shared vision.
- Common language between health professionals and ECE professionals.
- Understand and use what already exists for national competencies that have positive results. Don't reinvent the wheel. There is too much to do and we need implementation focus.
- We need to help educate parents about the importance of early years.
- Parents need support and education on child development.
- How to get pediatric providers and ECE providers to share and work together, not just side by side.
- Hospitals engagement in primary preventions supporting all parents in healthy child development.

- What is preventing school districts from investing in high-quality perks? Funding is an obvious challenge, but there are other known barriers for school districts. And how can these be addressed?
- Create partnerships with parents instead of a one-way knowledge relationship where trainers know everything and parents don't.
- What are the factors that led to scale (25 percent penetration) in "reach out and read," replication?
- How do we sustain efforts, beyond funding? Define this better.
- How do you connect the various health and ECE initiatives in communities? For example, ParentCorps and its three tiers is impressive—what else is going on in NYC and can connect to now?
- What interventions are successful at closing or minimizing inequities between populations regarding childhood achievement (beyond overall improvements)?
- Gaps of understanding the language between the various sectors that touch the lives of young children. Alignment so families feel supported in an integrated fashion.
- Peer-to-peer capacity building with parents and providers/teachers.
- More understanding about how parents are engaged outside of the provider setting.
- Role of environmental toxicants (e.g., heavy metals) in successful vocabulary development.
- Increase the communication between health/education sectors.
- How to scale when so much engagement of families requires the need to differentiate by method, content, format. Are there identified best practices in the field?
- Funding—how do we make this a priority for policy makers?
- On partnerships: what are the critical success factors for creating a multisector partnership?
- How do we help school systems see ECE and health care services?
- Support for translational efforts, technical assistance, and cross-sector training.

c. New insights (e.g., what you need to know about parents, teachers, caregivers)
   - What do parents want out of their ECE settings? Where is their voice?
   - As we move toward universal opportunity for pre-K, are the pre-K educators part of the public school system? Same criteria for hiring?
   - How do you define early care and education?

- How does the use of home care vary across the 0–5 age range?
- Are 60 percent of 6-month-olds in child care?
- Given focus on low income, are there lessons learned from mainstream (not economically challenged) that we should make sure is available to all, for equity?
- How are educational programs for ECE providers incorporating health into the curriculum?
- How can we honor and show respect for the people engaged in this work over decades of time?
- What is the evidence base regarding the costs of high-quality pre-K? To spread and scale, policy makers need to know general costs and cost-effectiveness (costs per outcomes gained).
- How are outcomes shared across sectors systematically?
- Does it ever undermine parenting confidence to offer programs that suggest they need assistance?
- What are the cultural norms of the families we are working with?
- Understand what families know about their child's development, and individualize from there to support developmentally appropriate information.
- Have we thought about grandparents as a trusted role model for parents and children?
- How can community health workers play a role?
- How can health care providers and systems help parents, caregivers?
- Approach to understanding of developmental delays.
- If we paid family members to stay home and care for 0–3 as a job, would that improve outcomes?
- Beyond outcomes regarding child achievement and wellness, what metrics matter to parents and caregivers regarding their own goals—use these when developing and evaluating programs, too.
- Are there ways we can encourage environmental supports to help families so they aren't making behavioral change (i.e., talking to baby) in a vacuum?
- What do working parents need to learn about spending time with their children?
- We have to hold families' culture at the center of our actions. This is hard and has to be revisited all the time.
- Status of parents/caregivers' mental health as it impacts their ability to care for their children.
- Do parents respond better to messages of preventing problems than meeting aspirations for their child? If no, what are implications for building awareness and buy-in?

- Parents need respectful culture-based engagement and mutual definitions of quality.
- Understand the risk factors [parents and caregivers] are experiencing and support the integration of a protective factors framework.
- Their own perspective of capacities to influence health—how can they truly co-create a system that promotes health?
- How are technology applications and tools impacting language and activity of young children? Are ECE providers aware of new or existing recommendations? How to communicate them?

Topic 2: Collaboration

a. How can we accelerate cross-sector collaboration in ECE and health? What do you need to help you and your organization collaborate effectively?
   - Leverage health sector requirements (e.g., CHNA) that can directly spark collaboration with other sectors, particularly as they relate to child health needs.
   - Nonprofit hospital community benefit is a $26 billion federal tax exemption.
   - How far would this go to close ECE equity gaps?
   - Resource redirection.
   - Getting funders to reallocate up front to gain better outcomes.
   - More opportunities for learning between early childhood education teachers and pediatricians.
   - Bridge the knowledge gap in both sectors.
   - Professional development conferences that are cross-sector.
   - Build ECE engagement with pediatric care into ACO quality metrics.
   - Honor the work that has been done over time that leads to where we are now.
   - Bring in as many perspectives as possible—together we are better!
   - Incentives, awareness, common motivation.
   - Regulations that are connected.
   - Incentives.
   - Training—not just usual suspects.
   - Use asset-based approach to leverage what's working and be willing to work in different ways together.
   - To collaborate with policy professionals and advocates, more attention and strategic thinking/planning needs to happen in regard to financing models.

- Funds and incentives work to redirect who is involved.
- Metrics can drive action and funding drive and link metrics.
- Streamlining of funding mechanisms.
- Shared approaches and objectives by main funders.

b. Main barriers to collaboration and the solutions to them?
- Lack of shared purpose and goals, not enough systems thinking.
- Competing agendas.
- There is an art and skill to learn how to do collaboration, especially across sectors.
- Lack of shared evaluation and mechanisms and data platforms.
- Upfront commitment to best possible goals and data-gathering processes. This maximizes outcomes and decreases level of needed investment in new data systems.
- Leadership commitment.
- Shared information and data.
- Lack of understanding perspectives, silos.
- Understanding the benefits and challenges for all partners.
- Are they effective? How do we measure how collaborations are affecting population-level outcomes?
- Takes more time that = more money. Few funders really support those costs.
- Turf.
- The complexities of the issues surrounding early childhood make it difficult to prioritize where public and private efforts should be focused.
- Lack of skills on how to build strong partnerships.
- Common language: agreed upon goals, metrics.
- Data sharing and alignment.
- Trust, history of working together.
- Funding systems tend to be siloed—fund collaborative teams.
- Core funding for integration functions.
- Silos, jargon, lack of personal relationships.
- Lack of funding.
- Need to have common grounding in theory and best practices in ECE.
- Independent goals, funders, strategic plans, metrics—must align in a true collaborative.
- Barriers: disconnected academic communities—solution: opportunities like today.

c. What have we learned from other cross-sector collaborations that could help to inform ECE/health interactions?
   - Intentionality; clear agreement on early outcomes and shared credit; leadership commitment.
   - Review ReThink Health Pathway Model.
   - Be open, understand that formal definitions of quality might not bring all who need to be at the table to the table.
   - Collaboration costs—need "glue" money.
   - Clear rules of engagement: bylaws, expectations, collective impact, buy-in—hard but critical.
   - Center for Work, Health, & Well-Being.
   - Cross-sector collaborations tend to be more effective than larger-scale ways to effect change.
   - Collaborative funding is key.
   - Make case about root cause to push many people together for collaboration.
   - Create small group of passionate leaders to drive and oversee the collaboration; leaders have to bring an equity lens.
   - You need clarity on the results and then identify shared measures and metrics.
   - Personal relationships are key: people make change.
   - The importance of partnering with community members at the program development stage → evolution in authentic, bi-directional way.
   - [Look at] Healthy Monadnock 2020.
   - Be the Change San Diego, ReThink Health Ventures; Atlanta Regional Collaboration for Health Improvement.
   - Relationships are key; start with small goals and wins; it takes time.
   - Partnerships and governance structures are key.
   - Who is at the table, and are they contributing?
   - How are they organized to do work, accountable for impact?
   - How are city, health systems structured and organized to support work, and are they active partners?
   - You need to be intentional, focused, and organized. Effective collaboration does not just happen.
   - Importance of anchor institutions.

d. New insights?
   - Let health sector take more of a leadership role in early childhood development system building 0–3.
   - There is more to sustainability than funding.
   - Rethink what is already in place, asset-based approach.

- 10:1 gap in eligibility: enrollment is shocking.
- Public–private partnerships and collaboration—get clarity on roles and levers in public sector versus private sector.
- We're doing similar work in ECE—how can we learn from each other, so we don't all need to "reinvent the wheel"?
- Lincoln, NE, is a great example of a holistic, community-driven approach.
- Building vocabulary can improve population health.
- ParentCorps resources.

Topic 3: Policy

a. What are the main policy levers that could support the spread/scale of health/ECE coordination?
    - Require hospital to use a percent of community benefit dollars to invest in ECE.
    - Developmental screening for all.
    - Strengthen focus on well-being and social emotional learning for workforce.
    - Specific for Paula—require 25 percent of nonprofit hospital tax advantage provided in each local area (but what about for profits?).
    - Developing competencies that elevate all without making caretaking inaccessible to those in our immigrant or low-income communities. Think access to providers that look/sound like me.
    - Cohort training models, cultural brokers, developed with the communities.
    - Universal pre-K.
    - Quality standards for providers.
    - Training for parents.
    - Nurse–family partnership and/or similar home visiting programs.
    - Need greater alignment of MCH and ECE.
    - Broaden advocacy base to unsuspecting partners, such as Fight Crime, Invest in Kids.

b. What policy actions can be taken to address some of the challenges in spreading and scaling effective early childhood care and education interventions and programs?
    - No more investments in new models; focus on scaling those we know work.
    - Health plans provide enhanced rates for implementation.
    - Centralized repository of evidence-based practices tied to health and education guidelines.

- Give funding for careful implementation and innovation not just evidence-based programs.
- Federal tax incentives.
- Engage national employers.
- Pay for value-based health care to drive ECE outcomes since all of the dollars are in health care—use these dollars to pay for what works in ECE.
- Requiring definitions of quality to be rooted in community values in addition to evidence-based practice so all will want to access high-quality care.
- Focus more on building capacity to teach practice in adults in settings other than evidence-based programs.
- Braided funding to support effective inclusion practices.
- Federal government provides technical assistance and support focused on prevention.
- Advocacy rooted in communities that builds demand for quality.

c. What needs to be done to support and increase investments for new ideas and innovation in early childhood care and education?
   - Focus on workforce and packaging what they need in evidence-based supports, including compensation.
   - Elevate best practices with public–private partnerships—look at tobacco or sugar-sweetened beverage taxes, tax credits, business champions for fundraising.
   - Create scorecards for each elected official's district/jurisdiction that includes reading by grade 3 by district/race/ethnicity/income; also graduation rates and link to early childhood education rates.
   - Training and education of health care providers at every level—undergrad, medical school, residency, and continuing education—should include exposure to role of early childhood care and education.
   - Get early childhood interventions (high-quality, accessible early care and learning) on radar of ACOs and hospitals and health systems before they move to value-based payment system.
   - Make the case; find start-up prevention dollars, show how money is saved, costs avoided through prevention to sustain and increase investments.
   - Health care and education—where money is in the system and sector that save when early childhood prevention is done well.
   - Need to explore how existing funds are being used to support ECE and health—look for duplication of effort.

- Ensure that business leaders and politicians understand the ROI in multiple budgets from ECE money.
- Don't assume that a rationale of benefit to children is sufficient.
- Use implementation science—performance evaluations more for learning, not just focus on outcomes.
- CMMI needs to release FOA on children.
- Establish economic developmental sequelae—cost to society.
- Frame the message and ask to speak to language/interest of different sectors.
- Think outside the "children's advocacy" silo.
- →research→advocacy→messaging→research, etc.
- Local community organizing.
- Understand how tax policy can be part of the answer.
- Include ECE in student funding formula for school.
- ECE and K–12 health systems—[public] health, pediatricians, and business *all* work together.

d. What policy actions can be taken to increase collaboration and synergies between those working in the health sector and the early childhood care and education sector?
   - Align, harmonize, or collaborate on community needs assessments both sectors do (see National Academies report *Communities in Action*).
   - Mandate screening in pediatrics for social determinants of health.
   - Have IRS-required attention to ECE as a part of every CHNA.
   - Absenteeism as common outcome.
   - Need the forums for conversation, engagement, and problem solving between and across sectors.
   - Link ACO and MIPS/MACRA quality metrics with early childhood care and education for pediatric visits.
   - Required ECE landscape assessment as part of CHNA.

D

Biographical Sketches of Workshop Speakers and Moderators[1]

George Askew, M.D., is the deputy commissioner of the New York City Department of Health and Mental Hygiene in the Division of Family and Child Health. He previously served as the first chief medical officer for the Administration for Children and Families (ACF) at the U.S. Department of Health and Human Services (HHS). In that role he provided expert advice and consultation to the assistant secretary for children and families on the development of plans, programs, policies, and initiatives that address the health needs and strengths of vulnerable children and families. Prior to this appointment, Dr. Askew served as senior policy advisor for early childhood health and development for ACF, where he led a team working on inter-departmental health-related early childhood initiatives and programs, including the home visiting program, joint Head Start and child care initiatives, and programs or initiatives administered and developed in coordination with other HHS agencies. During a previous stint at HHS, Dr. Askew served as the chief of the Health and Disabilities Services Branch of the Head Start Bureau and medical advisor to the Commissioner for the Administration on Children, Youth, and Families. He provided leadership in developing policies, oversight, and support systems to improve the quality of outcomes of medical, dental, nutritional, mental health, and disabilities services to Head Start and Early Head Start children and families. He is former deputy chief executive officer (CEO) of Voices for America's Children, the founder of Docs for Tots, former CEO

[1] † = member of the workshop planning committee; * = member of the roundtable.

and president of Jumpstart for Young Children, and a former epidemic intelligence service officer for the Centers for Disease Control and Prevention. As a child and family advocate, because of his initiative, vision, and national impact, Dr. Askew was selected as an Ashoka International Fellow. He was recognized as a national and global leader for his efforts to link health professionals with child advocacy, embodying the ideals of civic engagement and creative solution building nurtured by the international fellowship program. Born in Cleveland, Ohio, Dr. Askew was a Head Start graduate and later attended Harvard University and received a B.A. in psychology and social relations, emphasizing child development. He received his medical degree from the Case Western Reserve University School of Medicine.

Laurie Brotman, Ph.D., is the Bezos Family Foundation Professor of Early Childhood Development, a professor of population health and child and adolescent psychiatry, and the director of the Center for Early Childhood Health and Development at the New York University School of Medicine. Dr. Brotman recently completed an Ascend Fellowship in two-generation approaches to poverty reduction at the Aspen Institute. Throughout her career, Dr. Brotman has focused on strategies to promote health and development among young children living in low-income, urban communities. In a systematic series of randomized controlled trials with traditionally underserved and understudied racial and ethnic minority populations, Dr. Brotman and her research team have demonstrated that developmentally and theoretically informed family intervention can result in long-term benefits for children's behavior, mental health, physical health, and academic achievement. This work shows the potential impact of creating safe, nurturing, and predictable early environments at home and in the classroom and highlights the preschool period as a window of opportunity for promoting population health and reducing health disparities. Dr. Brotman has been funded by the National Institute for Mental Health and the Institute of Education Sciences over two decades to carry out this work. In 1998, Dr. Brotman and colleagues developed ParentCorps, a family-centered, culturally relevant enhancement to prekindergarten programs that aims to attenuate the effects of poverty and adverse childhood experiences on health and development. Building on two randomized controlled trials in 18 New York City (NYC) district schools with more than 1,200 children and families, Dr. Brotman and her team are currently partnering with the NYC Department of Education's Division of Early Childhood Education to scale, continuously improve, and rigorously evaluate ParentCorps programs, best practices, and tools throughout NYC's Pre-K for All system, which serves more than 70,000 4-year-olds annually. This work is supported by contracts with the New

York State Office of Mental Health and the NYC Department of Education and by grants from five family foundations. Dr. Brotman was named to the YWCA Academy of Women Leaders in 2009, served two terms on the board of directors of the Society for Prevention Research, and was chair of the society's 2015 annual meeting. Dr. Brotman was awarded the Society for Prevention Research's Community, Culture, and Prevention Science Award in 2009 and also the Cornell University College of Human Ecology's Distinguished Alumni Achievement Award in 2014.

Judith Carta, Ph.D., is the interim director of the Juniper Gardens Children's Project, a senior scientist in the Institute for Life Span Studies, and a professor of special education at the University of Kansas. She currently co-directs the national Bridging the Word Gap Research Network. Her science focuses on developing strategies to minimize the effects of poverty on children's outcomes and on developing practices that teachers and parents can use to promote children's language, early literacy, and social outcomes. Her key research and policy interests include advancing the quality of children's caregiving environments, methods for monitoring the progress of young children, and strategies for promoting family engagement in early intervention programs. She has been the principal investigator of several multi-site research projects and centers funded by the National Institutes of Health, the Institute of Educational Sciences, and the Administration for Children and Families. She was a member of the Federal Advisory Panel on Head Start Research and Evaluation and of the Division of Early Childhood's Commission on Recommended Practices, and she served as the editor of *Topics in Early Childhood Special Education*. She was the recipient of the 2016 Irvin Youngberg Research Award given to recognize an individual whose applied research has had significant impact and relevance to the state of Kansas.

Debbie Chang, M.P.H.,[†*] is the senior vice president of policy and prevention and a corporate officer for Nemours Children's Health System. Ms. Chang works to leverage Nemours's expertise and experience to spread and scale what works through national policy and practice changes to improve the health and well-being of children nationwide. In addition, Ms. Chang and her team work with internal leaders to build on and continue Nemours innovative transformation to a value-based health system. She also co-directs Moving Health Care Upstream, a national collaborative network to test, develop, and spread innovative population health strategies. She is the principal investigator of a $20 million, 5-year cooperative agreement with the Centers for Disease Control and Prevention (CDC) to improve healthy eating and physical activity for children from birth to age 5 years. Ms. Chang was the founding executive director of Nemours

Health and Prevention Services, an operating division devoted to using a comprehensive multisector, place-based model to improve children's health in Delaware. She serves on the National Academies' Board on Children, Youth, and Families and roundtables on Population Health and Improvement and Obesity Solutions; the National Center for Children in Poverty; the University of Michigan Griffith Leadership Center Board; the Asian and Pacific Islander Health Forum; and the Winter Park Health Foundation Board. Nemours is a founding member of the Partnership for a Healthier America and of the National Convergence Partnership, a unique collaboration of leading foundations focused on healthy people and healthy places. Ms. Chang has more than 29 years of federal and state government and private-sector experience in the health field. She has held key government positions, including deputy secretary of health care financing at the Maryland Department of Health and Mental Hygiene, with oversight for Maryland's Medicaid program, and the national director of the State Children's Health Insurance Program (SCHIP) when it was first implemented in 1997 at the U.S. Department of Health and Human Services. Ms. Chang's work on population health, child health systems transformation, Medicaid, SCHIP, and Nemours's prevention-oriented health system—including its CDC Pioneering Innovation award-winning statewide childhood obesity program—has been widely published. Ms. Chang holds a master's degree in public health policy and administration from the University of Michigan and a bachelor's degree in chemical engineering from the Massachusetts Institute of Technology.

Marquita F. Davis, Ph.D.,[†] is the deputy director for early learning on the Pacific Northwest team at the Bill and Melinda Gates Foundation. She most recently served as the executive director of the Jefferson County Committee for Economic Opportunity (JCCEO), a community action agency in Birmingham, Alabama. JCCEO believes that all people, regardless of their income or social status, are entitled to a life of decency and dignity. At JCCEO, Dr. Davis was responsible for running Head Start and pre-K centers, remaining grounded in the work of what teachers and center leaders are really doing day to day and what it takes to put young students on the path to success. Prior to joining the JCCEO in 2013, Dr. Davis served as the Alabama state finance director. She was appointed to the state finance post in 2011 and was the first female and second African American to hold the position. Dr. Davis previously served as a state commissioner of the Department of Children's Affairs overseeing statewide pre-K and as the director of the Alabama State Office of School Readiness, where she led efforts to gain legislative support for expansion of pre-K. She also worked for JCCEO from 2004 to 2008 as the director of child development services before she went to work for Governor Bob Riley's administration. She received a B.S. from Northern Illinois University, an M.S. from Alabama A&M University, and a Ph.D. from the University of Alabama at Birmingham in early childhood education and development.

Danielle Ewen, M.P.A., is a senior policy advisor at EducationCounsel, working to connect early childhood and K–12 systems at the federal, state, and local levels. Prior to this position, she served in numerous leadership positions in child care and early education policy. She previously served as the director of the Office of Early Childhood Education in the District of Columbia Public Schools (DCPS), where she oversaw the operations of programs serving 3- and 4-year-old children in high-quality, comprehensive classrooms. Prior to her work in DCPS, Ms. Ewen served as the director of the child care and early education team at the Center for Law and Social Policy (CLASP). At CLASP, she worked on federal and state issues around child care and early education, particularly the reauthorizations of the Child Care and Development Block Grant and Head Start.

Jennifer Frey, Ph.D.,[†] coordinates the Early Childhood Special Education Graduate Program in the Department of Special Education and Disability Studies and directs the Early Childhood Research Program in The George Washington University (GWU) Autism and Neurodevelopmental Disorders Institute (ANDI). Dr. Frey received her doctorate in education and human development with a major in special education and specializations in educational psychology and applied behavior analysis from Vanderbilt University. While a doctoral student, Dr. Frey was a Dunn Family Scholar of Educational and Psychological Assessment, and she received the Melvyn I. Semmel Dissertation Research Award. Dr. Frey also earned a master of education in early childhood special education and a bachelor of science, summa cum laude, in cognitive studies and child development from Peabody College of Vanderbilt University. Dr. Frey's research focuses on early language acquisition and partner-mediated approaches to early social communication interventions. She works with parents, teachers, and children across home, school, and clinic settings to examine the effects of naturalistic strategies used to support and enhance language and social behavioral development of young children with autism and other neurodevelopmental disorders, young children at risk for poor language and social emotional outcomes due to factors associated with cleft palate, and children at risk for learning challenges due to poverty-related risk factors. Dr. Frey is a member of the national Bridging the Word Gap Research Network: Work Group #1 (Interventions Designed for Parents) funded by the Health Resources and Services Administration of the U.S. Department of Health and Human Services and serves as a mentor to a Bridging the Word Gap Emerging Research Scholar. She also collaborates with GWU ANDI faculty on research investigating social learning, novel biomarkers of language development, and neural mechanisms that predict the success of social communication interventions for young children with autism. Her work has been published in leading journals and handbooks in the fields of special education, speech-language pathology, and school psychology. Dr. Frey, a recent nominee for the GWU Bender Teaching Award, also advises graduate students and teaches courses related to assessment of young children with special needs, language development and intervention, behavior management, research and trends in special education, and quantitative research methods. She is the principal investigator of the Voyages master's and graduate certificate in autism spectrum disorders personnel preparation grant and the LEEAD leadership grant, both funded by the U.S. Department of Education's Office of Special Education Programs, and she also serves as a center associate in the Center for Health and Health Care in Schools at the GWU Milken Institute School of Public Health.

Allison Gertel-Rosenberg, M.S., is the director of national prevention and practice for the Nemours National Office of Policy and Prevention. She is responsible for leading the office's efforts to spread and scale promising practices and strategic prevention initiatives designed to curb childhood obesity on a national scale and for initiatives that involve the intersection of population health and clinical care. These efforts have included the highly successful Let's Move! Child Care; Healthy Kids, Healthy Future; and the National Early Care and Education Learning Collaborative initiative with the Centers for Disease Control and Prevention. Ms. Gertel-Rosenberg's involvement has run the gamut from securing funding for these collaborations, as she has leveraged $47 million in grants over the course of her career, to playing a critical role in planning and implementing the strategic and operational measures necessary to make them successful. Ms. Gertel-Rosenberg received her M.S. in health policy and management from the Harvard School of Public Health and her B.S. in public health from Rutgers College.

Rolf Grafwallner, Ph.D., is the program director for early childhood initiatives at the Council of Chief State School Officers in Washington, DC, where he works with states to improve learning opportunities and outcomes for young children. Prior to joining the council, Dr. Grafwallner worked on early childhood policy and school reform as an assistant state superintendent at the Maryland State Department of Education. He was a teacher, program director, and administrator prior to joining the department. His expertise is in large-scale early childhood assessments, governance, finance, organizational leadership, and early education systems building. He received his Ph.D. from the University of Maryland, College Park, in education policy planning and administration.

Gloria Higgins has been the president of Executives Partnering to Invest in Children (EPIC) since September 6, 2012. Higgins has more than 30 years of experience in the financial services sector and has brought her private sector and civic engagement expertise to the organization, which works to harness the political and financial capital of Colorado's business leaders to ensure that all children develop into healthy, educated, and productive working adults. Ms. Higgins has a solid history leveraging multiple constituent commitments to improve early childhood programming. This is evidenced by her experience as the founding board chair for the Denver Preschool Program, which enhances the quality of early childhood education and access for all of Denver's 4-year-olds. For this role she was awarded Exceptional Board Volunteer in 2009. Ms. Higgins was involved in the founding of multiple businesses, including Higgins, Meritt & Higgins; Digital Partner; Epic Advisors, Inc.; and Ruby Ridge Insights LLC. The focus of each organization has been financial services for multi-generational families, blended with technology and financial data aggregation. Ms. Higgins has served on numerous business boards and advisory committees, including for Citywide Banks, Northstar Advisors, Innovest Portfolio Solutions, and the Wynkoop Brewery. She has also been active in the philanthropic and nonprofit community, including with the Colorado Children's Chorale, The Center for the Study of Taxation, Focus Points Family Resource Center, the Denver General Hospital Finance Committee, and the JFM Foundation. In 2010 she was acknowledged as a finalist in business and finance as one of Denver's Outstanding Women in Business by the *Denver Business Journal*.

George Isham, M.D., M.S.,* is a senior advisor to HealthPartners responsible for working with the board of directors and the senior management team on health and quality-of-care improvement for patients, members, and the community. Dr. Isham is also a senior fellow of the HealthPartners Research Foundation, and he facilitates progress at the intersection of population health research and public policy. Dr. Isham is active nationally and currently co-chairs the National Quality Forum–convened Measurement Application Partnership, chairs the clinical program committee of the National Committee for Quality Assurance (NCQA), and is a member of NCQA's committee on performance measurement. He is a former member of the Centers for Disease Control and Prevention's Task Force on Community Preventive Services and of the Agency for Health Care Quality's U.S. Preventive Services Task Force, and he currently serves on the advisory committee to the director of Centers for Disease Control and Prevention. His experience as a general internist was with the U.S. Navy at the Freeport Clinic in Freeport, Illinois, and as a clinical assistant professor of medicine at the University of Wisconsin Hospitals and Clinics in Madison, Wisconsin. In 2014 Dr. Isham was elected to the National Academy of Medicine. Dr. Isham is the chair of the Health and Medicine Division's (HMD's) Roundtable on Health Literacy and has chaired three studies in addition to serving on a number of HMD studies related to health and quality of care. In 2003 Dr. Isham was appointed as a lifetime national associate of the National Academy of Sciences in recognition of his contributions to the work of HMD.

Jacqueline Jones, Ph.D.,[†] is the president and chief executive officer of the Foundation for Child Development, where she is responsible for developing and implementing its strategic vision and goals. Prior to her tenure at the Foundation for Child Development, Dr. Jones served as a senior advisor on early learning to secretary of education Arne Duncan and as the country's first deputy assistant secretary for policy and early learning in the U.S. Department of Education. Prior to her position in the Obama administration, Dr. Jones served as the assistant commissioner for the Division of Early Childhood Education in the New Jersey State Department of Education and as a senior research scientist at the Educational Testing Service in Princeton for more than 15 years. Dr. Jones has been a visiting faculty member at the Harvard Graduate School of Education and a full-time faculty member at the City University of New York. She received her master's and Ph.D. degrees from Northwestern University.

Paula Lantz, Ph.D.,[†*] is the associate dean for academic affairs and a professor of public policy at the Gerald R. Ford School of Public Policy at the University of Michigan, where she is also a professor of health management and policy. Dr. Lantz, a social demographer, studies the role of public health in health care reform, clinical preventive services (such as cancer screening and prenatal care), and social inequalities in health. She is particularly interested in the role of health care versus broad social policy aimed at social determinants of health in reducing social disparities in health status. She is currently doing research regarding the potential of social impact bonds to reduce Medicaid expenditures. Dr. Lantz received an M.A. in sociology from Washington University, St. Louis, and an M.S. in epidemiology and a Ph.D. in sociology from the University of Wisconsin.

Sarah LeMoine, M.S., is a thought leader in early childhood professional development (PD) systems, with expertise in regulations and policy, systems development and change, and workforce leadership and diversity issues. She holds an M.S. in leadership and policy with extensive experience of more than 27 years ranging from direct service work to national-level research and writing, technical assistance (TA) and training, policy analysis, and advocacy. Ms. LeMoine is the co-director of the Professional Development and Workforce Innovations Department at Zero to Three (ZTT). Previously, she was the director for the National Center on Child Care Professional Development Systems and Workforce Initiatives at ZTT; the director of state workforce systems policy at the National Association for the Education of Young Children (NAEYC); the TA manager and information services manager for the National Child Care Information Center (NCCIC); and a research and TA associate at the Wheelock College Center for Career Development. Ms. LeMoine has authored and co-developed numerous PD systems publications and tools, including the Zero to Three Critical Competencies for Infant-Toddler Educators™; a PD system cost analysis tool; chapters in Teachers College Press–edited volumes on PD governance, competencies, and systems; NAEYC's and the National Association of Child Care Resource and Referral Agencies' Training and TA Glossary; NAEYC's Policy Blueprint; NCCIC's simplified systems model referred to as "the tree" and the related toolkit; and the first national TA paper on cross-sector PD systems.

Phyllis Meadows, Ph.D., MSN, RN,[†*] is a senior fellow in the health program at The Kresge Foundation engaging in all levels of grantmaking activity. Since joining The Kresge Foundation in 2009, she has advised the health team on the development of its overall strategic direction and provided leadership in the design and implementation of grantmaking initiatives and projects. Ms. Meadows has also coached team members and created linkages to national organizations and experts in the health field. In addition, she regularly reviews grant proposals, aids prospective grantees in preparing funding requests, and provides health-related expertise. Her 30-year career spans the nursing, public health, academic, and philanthropic sectors. She is the associate dean for practice at the University of Michigan's School of Public Health and has lectured at Wayne State University's School of Nursing, Oakland University's School of Nursing, and Marygrove College. From 2004 to 2009 Ms. Meadows served as the deputy director, director, and public health officer at the Detroit Department of Health and Wellness Promotion. In the early 1990s she traveled abroad as a Kellogg International Leadership Fellow and subsequently joined the W.K. Kellogg Foundation as a program director. She also served as director of nursing for The Medical Team–Michigan.

Larry Pasti, M.A.,[†] is a senior director at the Forum for Youth Investment. He provides support to communities and states interested in bringing the Ready by 21 strategies, solutions, and standards into their local work. Through strategic coaching, technical assistance, and tools he guides leader groups to understand the "nuts and bolts" of collective impact and other important systems-level work. He listens first before advising local leaders and helping them target their actions with examples from communities large and small, bringing a big picture perspective to the work. Mr. Pasti joined the forum in October 2008, having retired after many years at the New York State Office of Children and Family Services, where as a bureau director he supported strategic planning and applied research for the agency. Much of his work revolved around coordination and collaboration of government and community youth work—such as rolling out New York's Integrated County Planning Project and the Ready by 21 Quality Counts Initiative—and on developing quality assurance and evaluations of evidence-based programs, with an emphasis in the child welfare and juvenile justice systems. Mr. Pasti has helped other state agencies coordinate the use of evidence-based programs and build infrastructure to support those programs, and he has worked closely with such national organizations as Search Institute, RAND, and Child Trends. Mr. Pasti holds a bachelor of science degree in secondary education from Plattsburgh State University and a master of arts in criminal justice from Albany State University, both in New York. His early job as a probation officer has influenced his focus on families throughout his career.

Aly Richards is currently the chief executive officer of the Permanent Fund for Vermont's Children, a philanthropic organization founded in 2000 to promote access to affordable, high-quality early care and learning for all Vermont children. Prior to this role, Ms. Richards served as the deputy chief of staff and the director of intergovernmental affairs for Vermont Governor Peter Shumlin. In this position, Ms. Richards had leading roles in several of the Shumlin administration's efforts to support early childhood—including winning competitive federal Race to the Top Early Learning Challenge and Preschool Expansion grants totaling $70 million and supporting the passage of universal pre-K, making Vermont the first state in the country to offer 10 hours of publicly funded pre-K to all 3- and 4-year-olds. For her leadership, Ms. Richards was selected as a 2013 Toll Fellow by the Council of State Governments and as the 2014 Vermont Champion for Education by the New England Secondary School Consortium. Prior to joining the governor's office, Ms. Richards served on the 2008 Obama campaign and worked as the mid-Atlantic deputy finance director at the Democratic National Committee.

She received her B.A. with honors in international relations from Brown University. Ms. Richards also currently serves as a trustee of the Vermont State Colleges and lives in Montpelier, Vermont.

Krista Scott, M.S.S.W., is the senior director for Child Care Health Policy at Child Care Aware® of America. In her current role she is charged with supporting policy initiatives that make child care settings healthier communities for children and providers. Ms. Scott started her career in public service during college, where she worked for several nonprofit organizations that served youth in after school activities. She has experience working in Head Start/child care settings, providing disabilities services, mental health consultation, and family services. She also has many years working in state special education and disabilities programs, working toward creating inclusive environments and ensuring that services are delivered in accordance with federal law. Ms. Scott has her bachelor's degree in political science and her M.S.S.W. with a focus on management and policy.

Kimberly Shinn-Brown has a B.S. degree in early childhood education and elementary education from the University of Alabama and has invested 23 years with Ozarks Area Community Action Corporation (OACAC) Head Start in a variety of positions, all of which centered on partnering with families with young children. For the past 10 years, she has been the program director for OACAC Head Start, responsible for strategic planning, community partnership development, and grants management for the agency, which serves nearly 1,000 low-income children and families across 10 counties in southwest Missouri. She has been recognized as one of Springfield's 40 Under 40 and is a University of California, Los Angeles–Johnson & Johnson Head Start Management Fellow.

Michelle Suarez, M.Ed., is an early childhood developer for Prosper Lincoln. Ms. Suarez is a lifelong educator whose career has been spent serving the most vulnerable children and families. Ms. Suarez retired as a 19-year Lincoln Public Schools elementary principal (Calvert and Everett). Before becoming an administrator, she taught preschool, kindergarten, first grade, and sixth grade over 15 years in three school districts. Throughout her public school career, Ms. Suarez specialized in parent engagement and community partnership to support strong schools. She earned her bachelor's degree in elementary education and her master's degree in educational administration from the University of Nebraska–Lincoln.

Valora Washington, Ph.D.,[†] is the chief executive officer of the Council for Professional Recognition. In her career Dr. Washington has co-created several institutions, such as Michigan's Children, a statewide advocacy group; the Early Childhood Funders Collaborative; and The CAYL Institute. Frequently tapped for senior-level service, she has been the co-chair of the Massachusetts Governor's School Readiness Commission; board chair for Voices for America's Children; secretary of the National Association for the Education of Young Children (NAEYC); chair of the Black Caucus of the Society for Research in Child Development; co-chair of the National Head Start Association Commission on 2010; and a member of numerous task forces and boards, including of the Boston Children's Museum and Wheelock College. Prior to founding The CAYL Institute in 2003, Dr. Washington was the chief executive officer of the Unitarian Universalist Service Committee and vice president of the Kellogg Foundation. She has held executive and tenured teaching positions at institutions including Antioch College and the University of North Carolina at Chapel Hill. Since 2001 she has been a certified association executive with the American Society of Association Executives. Committed to action research and policy change, she is a co-author or co-editor of more than 50 publications, including *Children of 2010, Children of 2020, Ready or Not: Leadership Choices in Early Care and Education*, and *Role, Relevance and Reinvention: Higher Education and Early Care and Education*. Examples of effective advocacy include work to change the voucher system in Massachusetts that resulted in 52,000 children having opportunities for a 1-year certification period. Designing and coordinating efforts to change the child welfare system in 13 states, the Families for Kids initiative is regarded as leading to important legislative changes enacted by President Clinton. Among many honors, she holds honorary doctorate degrees from both Bennett College and Meadville Lombard Theological School. She was selected for the prestigious Barr Fellowship in 2009. Professional recognition has been received from Boston AEYC; NAEYC Black Caucus; Cambridge Resource and Referral Agency; Center for Adoption Research, University of Massachusetts; National Association of Black Social Workers; United Way of Massachusetts Bay; and others. She was named one of "25 most Influential Working Mothers" by *Working Mother* magazine in February 1997 and one of Ten Outstanding Young Women of America from 62,000 nominations in 1980. She was educated at both Indiana University and Michigan State University.

Marcy Whitebook, Ph.D., directs the Center for the Study of Child Care Employment at the Institute for Research on Labor and Employment at the University of California, Berkeley, which she founded in 1999. Her research focuses on issues of compensation, work environments, and appropriate and accessible professional preparation for the early childhood workforce, with specific attention to how these issues relate to children's development and learning. Her most recent reports—the *2016 Early Childhood Workforce Index* and *Worthy Work, STILL Unlivable Wages: The Early Care and Education Workforce 25 Years After the National Child Care Staffing Study*—document the current status of the workforce and analyze how federal and state workforce policies serve to support or undermine effective teaching and contribute to inequitable services for children and families and often pose risks to the personal and familial well-being of the workforce itself. Prior to her current position, Dr. Whitebook was the founding executive director of the Washington-based Center for the Child Care Workforce, an organization she began in 1977 as the Child Care Employee Project. Dr. Whitebook has led several large-scale early childhood research projects, including the landmark 1989 National Child Care Staffing Study, which first brought public attention to the low wages and high turnover of child care teachers and the effect of these factors on child outcomes Dr. Whitebook earned her bachelor's degree in religious studies and master's degree in early childhood education from the University of California, Berkeley, and her Ph.D. in development studies in education from the University of California, Los Angeles. She began her career as an infant–toddler and preschool teacher.

Jodi Whiteman, M.Ed., is the co-director of professional development and workforce innovations for Zero to Three. In this position Ms. Whiteman is responsible for advancing Zero to Three's capacity to offer high-quality professional development and technical assistance services to the early childhood field. Ms. Whiteman serves as the project director for many grant-funded projects as well as private contracts housed in the professional development department. She has a wealth of experience providing professional development and technical assistance on a variety of early childhood topics nationally and internationally. Her past experiences as adjunct faculty at the Graduate School of Education at George Mason University, a bilingual speech/language therapist assistant, an infant/toddler child care director, an early intervention specialist, and a certified educator of infant massage inform her work. She has authored many professional articles on a variety of early childhood topics. Ms. Whiteman holds a B.S. in speech and hearing sciences from the University of Arizona and an M.Ed. in curriculum and instruction from George Mason University.